The Complete Alkaline Diet Guidebook for Beginners:

Understand pH & Eat Well with 50 Delicious & Easy Alkaline Recipes and a 10 Day Meal Plan

Contents

Chapter 1. Alkaline Basics

What is the Alkaline Diet?

The alkaline diet is still up for debate today regarding its possible impact on human health. Further research was conducted recently to highlight positive results and the diet showed some notable improvements in health conditions for many people.

This diet plan basically tasks you to eat alkaline forming food while limiting or eliminating acid forming food. Proponents of this diet suggest that your gut system has a particular alkaline environment, especially within the intestine where most of the digestion and absorption takes place. Therefore, alkaline food can help maintain that environment and improve enzyme production and function which also thrive in alkaline conditions. The concept of alkaline food, its impact, and in-depth details are further discussed in later chapters.

What is pH?

Substances are divided chemically into two broad categories based on the number of hydrogen ions present in them. Those with the highest number of ions have the lowest pH values, and are called Acids while those with the lower number of ions are Alkaline and have higher pH values. A scale was developed to measure the degrees of acidity and alkalinity of the substances. The scale ranges from 0 to 14 with acids falling between the 0 to 6 range, 7 being neutral, and alkalines (also known as base substances) falling between 8 and 14 in pH value. To test the pH values of food or other substances, a specific paper is used to identify the pH properties through colors. This is known as a litmus test.

How Food Affects Your Body

"We are what we eat." This axiom pretty much explains everything about the role of food in our life. It's not all about gaining energy and calories. Most food can offer that but gaining clean energy without toxins and other harmful elements is the goal here. When food breaks down it releases energy along with other compounds and elements that diffuse into your blood and function within the internal environment of the body, and influence all the metabolic processes. Food that can support these processes and maintain an optimum internal environment can make you healthy and physically fit. When the opposite happens, you may have health problems like poor sleep habits, weight gain, acid-related issues, weak bones, dehydration, mental illnesses, low metabolic activity, high cholesterol, diabetes, cancer, and many other diseases. This makes choosing the food you eat that much more important.

Why the Alkaline Diet Helps

Your body's enzymes, hormones, and microbiome work at an optimum alkaline pH level in most parts of the body. Acidic food does not only disrupt the internal environment of your gut, but the low pH levels transfer to your blood and organs. Everything from liver bile to pancreatic enzymes, saliva enzymes, gut bacteria, and blood enzymes and hormones need this alkalinity to function well. When you eat acidic food, the enzymes and bacteria can't work to break down the macronutrients in the food and they go undigested. That is where the alkaline diet helps.

Proof that the Alkaline Diet is Useful

Where many people consider the alkaline diet to be a myth or a far-fetched idea, Gerry K. Schwalfenberg studied the impact of the alkaline diet on various health aspects including bone strength, the ratio of ions for nerve impulses, hormonal growth, back pain, and cancer prevention. He found that those aspects were positively affected by increasing the amount of alkaline food in a diet. He also found that an alkaline environment allows chemotherapeutic agents to work successfully in cancer patients.

The Microbiome and its Role in Alkalinity

Your gut is home to millions of microbes that create a microbiome. These microbes help in digestion by releasing their own enzymes and breaking down micro and macronutrients. The by-products released by the microbes during digestion keeps the internal gut environment alkaline as it needs to be. All acid-producing food can disrupt this and, therefore, aid in killing beneficial gut bacteria. Alkaline food can help in this regard and help the microbes function properly.

The Ratio of Macros and How it Affects Alkalinity

Macronutrients including carbohydrates, proteins, and fat have different chemical compositions; some more acidic than others. For example, proteins have amino acids and complex amino acids are abundantly present in red meat which causes acidity. Most carbohydrates are, generally, less acidic, but complex carbs and foods high in carbs are more acidic and need to be avoided. Fats are a rich source of fatty acids that can negatively affect the alkalinity of the body and animal fat is completely restricted on the alkaline diet.

Chapter 2. How to Follow the Alkaline Diet

Health Conditions Improved by Eating a More Alkaline Diet

The alkaline diet is proven to be most effective in treating the following health issues:

- Insomnia
- Arthritis
- Muscle Pain
- Cancer
- Diabetes
- Bloating
- Gout

Alkaline Water

To aid the alkalinization of the internal body environment, alkaline food is not enough; alkaline water can also be added to your diet. Normal water is almost neutral in composition, whereas alkaline water is prepared by adding gut-friendly compounds that turn the water more alkaline. It is an easy way to incorporate something alkaline into your diet even when you are not eating. This water has a pH of 8 to 9. It is also used when the acid level in blood or urine is too severe in order to bring their values back to normal.

Alkaline Diet Frequently Asked Questions

Q. What is the relation between alkaline food and acid reflux?

Alkaline food is a good way to reduce the severity of the condition slightly by maintaining the pH level of your gut. Yet a diet completely specific to acid reflux treatment differs from the alkaline diet discussed in this book

Q. How can alkaline food help you lose weight?

To turn a diet more alkaline, there are several foods that need to be omitted including sugars, complex carbohydrates, beans, and grains. Eliminating these types of foods can help you lose weight.

Q. Does cooking affect the alkalinity and acidity of food?

No, that is actually not true. The chemical composition of food does not change in a way that could affect the acidity or alkalinity of them. Cooking might change the form of the food but not the pH value.

Alkaline- and Acid-Forming Foods

Foods that can reduce the pH of your entire gut or digestive system are called acid-forming foods while foods that make your gut pH level higher are known as alkaline-forming foods.

Acid-Forming Foods

Here is a list of all the acid-forming foods that are in a typical diet:

- Rice (white, brown, or basmati)
- Cheese

- Pasta
- Wheat germ
- Alcoholic drinks
- All meat (beef, pork, lamb, fish, and chicken)
- Mustard
- Ketchup
- Coffee and other caffeinated drinks
- Soy sauce
- Popcorn
- Mayonnaise
- White vinegar
- Nutmeg
- Tobacco
- Cornmeal, rye
- Colas
- Sweetened yogurt
- Refined table salt

Alkalinizing Foods

Here is a detailed list of alkalizing foods:

- Whey
- Plain yogurt
- Fruit juices
- Most herbal teas
- Garlic
- All vegetable juices
- Cayenne pepper
- Fresh, unsalted butter
- Peas
- Arrowroot flour

- Beans (green, soy, lima, and snap)
- Unsprouted sesame
- Potatoes
- Grains (flax, millet, quinoa, and amaranth)
- Nuts (almonds, pine, fresh coconut, and chestnuts)
- Miso
- Most vegetables
- Unprocessed sea salt
- Most spices
- Vanilla extract
- Sprouted seeds (alfalfa, radish, and chia)
- Gelatin
- Sweeteners like raw, unpasteurized honey, dried sugar cane juice (Sucanat), brown rice syrup
- Most herbs
- Brewer's yeast

Chapter 3. What Can and Cannot be Affected by What You Eat

Understanding the Difference between Blood pH, Saliva pH, and Urine pH

Blood pH

The measure of blood's pH level is vital as it can tell you about the entire internal environment of your human body. Its normal value ranges between 7.35 and 7.45 which is more neutral.

Urine pH

Acidic urine is concerning because its normal pH value should be between 6 and 7.5 which is close to neutral. Higher acidity means the body is dehydrating and producing more acidic elements which are entering the kidneys through the blood.

Saliva pH

Saliva is produced in the mouth and has many digestive enzymes responsible for its particular pH level. Human saliva has a normal pH level of 5.6 to 7.9 in value. This means it has to be slightly acidic to neutral in order to digest simple carbs and proteins.

Testing Urine and Saliva pH Levels

The pH of both urine and saliva can be tested at home with different acid testing strips. Saliva testing strips are easily available but don't eat anything at all for about 2 hours before this test as it might affect the natural pH of the saliva in your mouth. Take a cotton swab and roll its head in your mouth then drop the saliva over a strip. Check the colors and use the given scale on the box to detect the true pH value of your saliva. Use the same techniques with a litmus strip to check the pH of your urine. Put your sample in a small container and dap the strip with a few drops of urine and leave it for few minutes. Once the color appears, match it to the box and check the pH value. If the pH is far from neutral, then this can be concerning. In that case, consult your health physician and discuss the results and consider altering your diet accordingly.

The 80/20 Rule

The 80/20 rule is a frequently used rule when it comes to food. This rule can also be applied to the alkaline diet by keeping the food in your diet 80 percent alkaline and 20 percent acidic, you can enjoy the taste and it won't affect your health too much. This simple rule gives you a rough estimate of how an alkaline diet can be maintained. It saves you from completely restricting your diet and gives you a little window for mistakenly eating low-grade acidic food to some extent.

Fermented Foods and Their Role

The role of fermentation is to break down food and release certain byproducts. Fermented foods are rich in microbes, healthy and easily digestible nutrients great for your gut microbiome. Common fermented foods include tempeh, miso, sauerkraut, and kefir. The advantages of eating fermented foods are good digestion and improved gut health. These foods are also easier to keep and last longer than others with or without the refrigerator.

Alkaline Foods to Enjoy

Vegetables	Nuts and Spices	Fruits	Beverages	Oils and Dairy	Bread and grains
Asparagus	Chestnuts	Blackberries	Mineral water	Ghee	Oatmeal
Celery	Sea salt	Strawberries	Ginger tea	Olive oil	Apple crisp
Artichokes	Ginger root	Raspberries	Grapefruit juice	Avocado oil	Granola
Collard greens	Pumpkin seeds	Cantaloupe	Apple juice	Coconut oil	
Kale	Black pepper	Watermelon	Pineapple juice	Cod liver oil	
Endive	Cashews	Raisins	Grape juice		
Sweet potatoes	Garlic	Blueberries	Green tea		
Potato	Almonds	Apples			
Bell peppers	Cinnamon	Apricots			
Broccoli	Soy sauce	Avocado			
Cabbage		Banana			
Carrots					
Snow peas					
Cucumbers					
Cauliflower					
Brussels sprouts					

Chapter 4. Alkaline Diet Recipes

Breakfast Recipes

Nut & Seed Granola

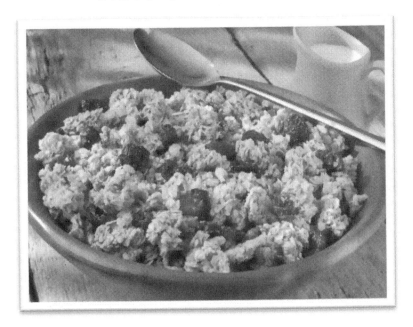

Preparation time: 15 minutes. **Cooking time:** 28 minutes. **Total time:** 43 minutes. **Servings:** 8

Ingredients:

- ½ cup unsweetened coconut flakes
- 1 cup raw almonds
- 1 cup raw cashews
- ¼ cup raw sunflower seeds, shelled
- ¼ cup raw pumpkin seeds, shelled

- ¼ cup coconut oil
- ½ cup maple syrup
- 1 tsp vanilla extract
- ½ cup golden raisins
- ½ cup black raisins
- Sea salt, to taste

How to Prepare:

1. Preheat the oven to 275 F. Line a large baking sheet with parchment paper.
2. In a food processor, add the coconut flakes, almonds, cashews, and seeds and pulse until chopped finely.
3. Meanwhile, in a medium non-stick pan, add the oil, maple syrup, and vanilla extract and cook for 3 minutes over medium-high heat stirring continuously.
4. Remove from the heat and immediately stir in the nut mixture.
5. Transfer the mixture to the prepared baking sheet and spread it out evenly.
6. Bake for about 25 minutes, stirring twice.
7. Remove the pan from the oven and immediately stir in the raisins.
8. Sprinkle with a little salt.
9. With the back of a spatula, flatten the surface of the mixture.
10. Set aside to cool completely.
11. Then, break into even chunks.
12. Serve with your choice of non-dairy milk and fruit topping.
13. For preserving, transfer this granola to an airtight container and keep it in the refrigerator.

Nutritional Values: Calories 382; Total Fat 25 g; Saturated Fat 9.6 g; Cholesterol 0 mg; Sodium 39 mg; Total Carbs 37.9 g; Fiber 3.5 g; Sugar 24 g; Protein 7.3 g

Chia Seed Pudding

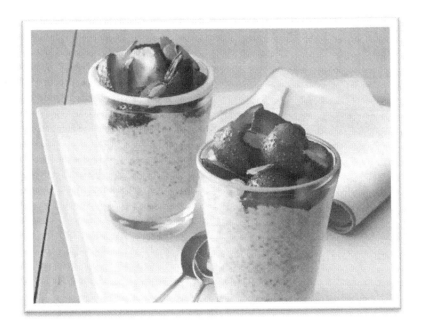

Preparation time: 10 minutes. **Total time:** 10 minutes.

Servings: 2

Ingredients:

- 1 cup unsweetened almond milk
- 1/3 cup chia seeds
- 1 tsp vanilla liquid stevia
- 1 tsp organic vanilla extract
- Pinch of sea salt
- ¼ cup fresh strawberries, hulled and sliced

How to Prepare:

1. Place all the ingredients except the strawberries in a bowl and whisk them until well combined.
2. Refrigerate the mixture for at least 10 minutes before serving.
3. Top the mixture with strawberry slices and serve.

Nutritional Values: Calories 218; Total Fat 13.8 g; Saturated Fat 0.2 g; Cholesterol 0 mg; Sodium 207 mg; Total Carbs 21.3 g; Fiber 16.9 g; Sugar 1.2 g; Protein 8.6 g

Buckwheat Porridge

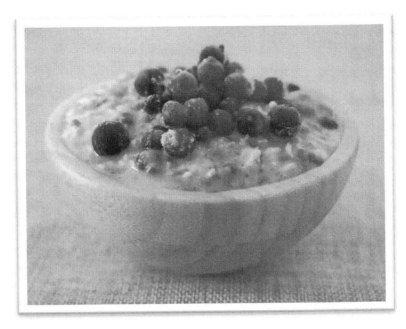

Preparation time: 10 minutes. **Total time:** 10 minutes.

Servings: 4

Ingredients:

- 2 cups buckwheat groats, soaked overnight and rinsed well
- 1½ cups unsweetened almond milk
- 2 tbsp chia seeds
- 1 tsp organic vanilla extract
- ¼ cup agave nectar
- 1 tsp ground cinnamon
- Pinch of sea salt
- ½ cup mixed fresh berries

How to Prepare:

1. Place the buckwheat groats, almond milk, chia seeds and vanilla extract in a food processor and pulse until well combined.
2. Add the agave nectar, cinnamon, and salt and pulse until smooth.
3. Transfer the mixture into serving bowls and serve immediately topped with berries.

Nutritional Values: Calories 325; Total Fat 5.5 g; Saturated Fat 0.5 g; Cholesterol 0 mg; Sodium 133 mg; Total Carbs 65.3 g; Fiber 11.3 g; Sugar 18 g; Protein 9.6 g

Spiced Quinoa Porridge

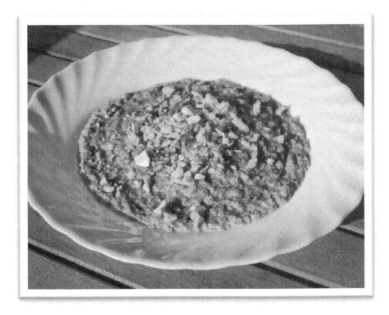

Preparation time: 10 minutes. **Cooking time:** 15 minutes. **Total time:** 25 minutes. **Servings:** 4

Ingredients:

- 1 cup uncooked red quinoa, rinsed and drained
- 2 cups water
- ½ tsp organic vanilla extract
- ½ cup coconut milk
- ¼ tsp fresh lemon peel, grated finely
- 10-12 drops liquid stevia
- 1 tsp ground cinnamon
- ½ tsp ground ginger
- ½ tsp ground nutmeg
- Pinch of ground cloves
- ¼ cup almonds, chopped

How to Prepare:

1. In a large pan, mix together the quinoa, water, and vanilla extract over medium heat and bring it to a boil.
2. Reduce the heat to low and simmer covered for about 15 minutes or until all the liquid is absorbed, stirring occasionally.
3. Add the coconut milk, lemon peel, stevia, and spices to the same pan and stir everything to combine.
4. Immediately, remove the pan from the heat and fluff the quinoa with a fork.
5. Divide the quinoa mixture into serving bowls evenly.
6. Top with almonds and serve.

Nutritional Values: Calories 265; Total Fat 12.8 g; Saturated Fat 6.9 g; Cholesterol 0 mg; Sodium 11 mg; Total Carbs 31.1 g; Fiber 4.8 g; Sugar 1.4 g; Protein 8 g

Fruity Oatmeal

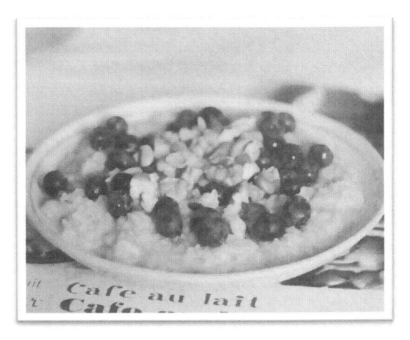

Preparation time: 10 minutes. **Total time:** 10 minutes.

Servings: 2

Ingredients:

- 1 cup rolled oats
- 1 large banana, peeled and mashed
- ¼ cup pecans, chopped
- 2 tsp chia seeds
- 1 cup unsweetened almond milk
- ¼ cup fresh blueberries
- 2 tbsp pecans, chopped

How to Prepare:

1. Place all the ingredients except the pecans in a large bowl and mix until well combined.
2. Refrigerate, covered overnight.
3. In the morning, remove the mixture from the refrigerator and serve it topped with almonds.

Nutritional Values: Calories 454; Total Fat 25.1 g; Saturated Fat 2.6 g; Cholesterol 0 mg; Sodium 93 mg; Total Carbs 53 g; Fiber 11.7 g; Sugar 11.5 g; Protein 10.6 g

Baked Oatmeal

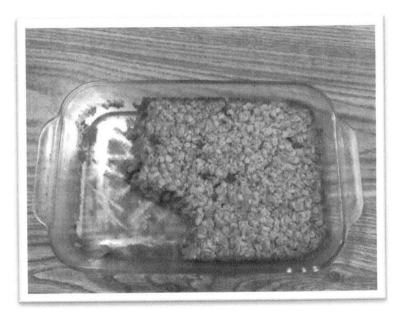

Preparation time: 15 minutes. **Cooking time:** 45 minutes. **Total time:** 1 hour. **Servings:** 6

Ingredients:

- 3 tbsp water
- 1 tbsp flax seed meal
- 3 cups unsweetened almond milk
- ¼ cup agave nectar
- 2 tbsp coconut oil, melted and cooled
- 2 tsp organic vanilla extract
- 1 tsp organic baking powder
- 1 tsp ground cinnamon
- ¼ tsp sea salt
- 2 cups old-fashioned rolled oats
- ½ cup pecans, chopped

28

How to Prepare:

1. In a bowl, add the water and flax seed meal and beat until well combined.
2. Set aside.
3. Place the flax seed mixture, almond milk, agave nectar, coconut oil, vanilla extract, baking powder, cinnamon, and salt in a large bowl and beat until well combined.
4. Add the oats and pecans and stir to combine.
5. Place the oat mixture into a lightly greased 8x8-inch and spread it into an even layer.
6. Cover the baking dish with plastic wrap and refrigerate for at least 8 hours or overnight.
7. Arrange a rack in the middle position of the oven and preheat the oven to 350 degrees F.
8. Remove the baking dish from the refrigerator and remove the plastic wrap.
9. With a spoon, stir the oat mixture well.
10. Bake uncovered for about 45 minutes or until the center is set.
11. Remove it from the oven and set it aside to cool slightly.
12. Serve warm with your desired toppings.

Nutritional Values: Calories 286; Total Fat 15.8 g; Saturated Fat 5.2 g; Cholesterol 0 mg; Sodium 17 mg; Total Carbs 32.8 g; Fiber 5.6 g; Sugar 10.9 g; Protein 5.4 g

Blueberry Pancakes

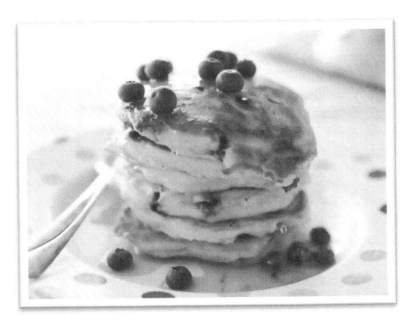

Preparation time: 10 minutes. **Cooking time:** 15 minutes. **Total time:** 25 minutes. **Servings:** 3

Ingredients:

- 1 cup rolled oats
- 1 medium banana, peeled and mashed
- ¼-½ cup unsweetened almond milk
- 1 tbsp organic baking powder
- 1 tbsp organic apple cider vinegar
- 1 tbsp agave nectar
- ½ tsp organic vanilla extract
- ½ cup fresh blueberries

How to Prepare:

1. Place all the ingredients except the blueberries in a large bowl and mix until well combined.
2. Gently fold in the blueberries.
3. Set the mixture aside for about 5-10 minutes.
4. Preheat a large non-stick skillet over medium-low heat.
5. Add about ¼ cup of the mixture and spread in an even layer.
6. Immediately, cover the skillet and cook for about 2-3 minutes or until golden.
7. Flip the pancake over and cook for 1-2 minutes more.
8. Repeat with the remaining mixture.
9. Serve warm.

Nutritional Values: Calories 183; Total Fat 2.3 g; Saturated Fat 0.4 g; Cholesterol 0 mg; Sodium 22 mg; Total Carbs 38.9 g; Fiber 4.9 g; Sugar 12.6 g; Protein 4.3 g

Tofu & Mushroom Muffins

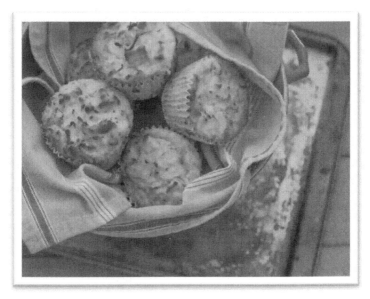

Preparation time: 15 minutes. **Cooking time:** 30 minutes. **Total time:** 45 minutes. **Servings:** 6

Ingredients:

- 1 tsp olive oil
- 1½ cups fresh mushrooms, chopped
- 1 scallion, chopped
- 1 tsp garlic, minced
- 1 tsp fresh rosemary, minced
- Freshly ground black pepper, to taste
- 1 (12.3 oz) package lite firm silken tofu, pressed and drained
- ¼ cup unsweetened soy milk
- 2 tbsp nutritional yeast
- 1 tbsp arrowroot starch
- 1 tsp coconut oil, softened
- ¼ tsp ground turmeric

How to Prepare:

1. Preheat oven to 375 degrees F. Grease a 12-cup muffin pan.
2. In a non-stick skillet, heat the oil over medium heat and sauté the scallions and garlic for about 1 minute.
3. Add the mushrooms and sauté for about 5-7 minutes.
4. Stir in the rosemary and black pepper and remove from the heat.
5. Set aside to cool slightly.
6. In a food processor, add the tofu and remaining ingredients and pulse until smooth.
7. Transfer the tofu mixture to a large bowl.
8. Fold in the mushroom mixture.
9. Transfer the mixture into the prepared muffin cups evenly.
10. Bake for about 20-22 minutes or until the tops become golden brown.
11. Remove the muffin pan from the oven and place it onto a wire rack to cool for about 10 minutes.
12. Carefully, invert the muffins onto a platter and serve warm.

Nutritional Values: Calories 87; Total Fat 3.7 g; Saturated Fat 1.1 g; Cholesterol 0 mg; Sodium 32 mg; Total Carbs 7.4 g; Fiber 1.8 g; Sugar 2.3 g; Protein 8 g

Eggless Tomato "Omelet"

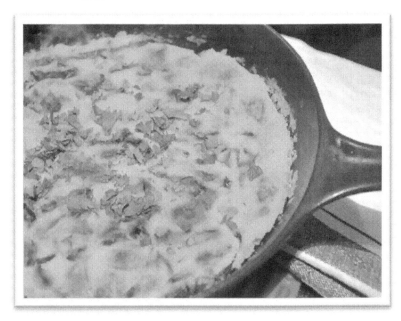

Preparation time: 15 minutes. **Cooking time:** 12 minutes. **Total time:** 27 minutes. **Servings:** 4

Ingredients:

- 1 cup chickpea flour
- ¼ tsp ground turmeric
- ¼ tsp red chili powder
- Pinch of ground cumin
- Pinch of sea salt
- 1½-2 cups water
- 1 medium onion, chopped finely
- 2 medium tomatoes, chopped finely
- 1 jalapeño pepper, chopped finely
- 2 tbsp fresh cilantro, chopped
- 2 tbsp olive oil, divided

How to Prepare:

1. In a large bowl, add the flour, spices, and salt and mix well.
2. Slowly, add the water and mix until well combined.
3. Fold in the onion, tomatoes, green chili, and cilantro.
4. In a large non-stick frying pan, heat ½ tablespoon of the oil over medium heat.
5. Add ½ of the tomato mixture and tilt the pan to spread it.
6. Cook for about 5-7 minutes.
7. Place the remaining oil over the "omelet" and carefully flip it over.
8. Cook for about 4-5 minutes or until golden brown.
9. Repeat with the remaining mixture.

Nutritional Values: Calories 267; Total Fat 10.3 g; Saturated Fat 1.3 g; Cholesterol 0 mg; Sodium 86 mg; Total Carbs 35.7 g; Fiber 10.2 g; Sugar 8.3 g; Protein 10.6 g

Quinoa Bread

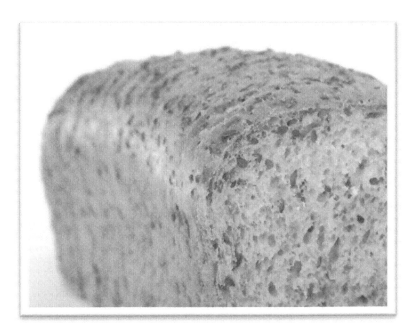

Preparation time: 10 minutes. **Cooking time:** 1½ hours. **Total time:** 1 hour 40 minutes. **Servings:** 12

Ingredients:

- 1¾ cups uncooked quinoa, soaked overnight, rinsed and drained
- ¼ cup chia seeds, soaked in ½ cup of water overnight
- ½ tsp bicarbonate soda
- Sea salt, to taste
- ¼ cup olive oil
- ½ cup water
- 1 tbsp fresh lemon juice

How to Prepare:

1. Preheat oven to 320 degrees F. Line a loaf pan with parchment paper.
2. Add all the ingredients in a food processor and pulse for about 3 minutes.
3. Place the mixture into the prepared loaf pan evenly.
4. Bake for about 1½ hours or until a toothpick inserted in the center comes out clean.
5. Remove it from the oven and place the loaf pan onto a wire rack to cool for at least 10-15 minutes.
6. Carefully, invert the bread onto the rack to cool completely before slicing.
7. With a sharp knife, cut the bread loaf into desired sized slices and serve.

Nutritional Values: Calories 151; Total Fat 7.2 g; Saturated Fat 0.8 g; Cholesterol 0 mg; Sodium 21 mg; Total Carbs 18.3 g; Fiber 3.8 g; Sugar 0 g; Protein 4.5 g

Lunch Resipes

Tomato & Greens Salad

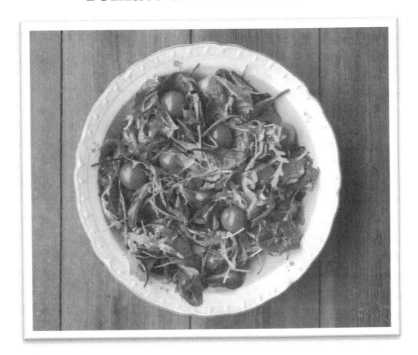

Preparation time: 15 minutes. **Total time:** 15 minutes.
Servings: 4

Ingredients:

- 6 cups fresh baby greens
- 2 cups cherry tomatoes
- 2 scallions, chopped
- 2 tbsp extra-virgin olive oil
- 2 tbsp fresh orange juice
- 1 tbsp fresh lemon juice

How to Prepare:

1. Place all the ingredients in a large bowl and toss to coat well.
2. Cover the bowl and refrigerate for about 6-8 hours.
3. Remove from the refrigerator and toss well before serving.

Nutritional Values: Calories 88; Total Fat 7.2 g; Saturated Fat 1.1 g; Cholesterol 0 mg; Sodium 11 mg; Total Carbs 5.9 g; Fiber 1.8 g; Sugar 3.8 g; Protein 1.5 g;

Strawberry & Apple Salad

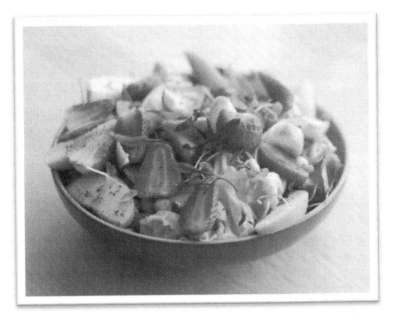

Preparation time: 15 minutes. **Total time:** 15 minutes.

Servings: 4

Ingredients:

For Salad:

- 4 cups mixed lettuce, torn
- 2 apples, cored and sliced
- 1 cup fresh strawberries, hulled and sliced
- ¼ cup pecans, chopped

For Dressing:

- 3 tbsp apple cider vinegar
- 3 tbsp olive oil
- 1 tbsp agave nectar
- 1 tsp poppy seeds

How to Prepare:

1. For the salad, place all the ingredients in a large bowl and mix well.
2. For the dressing, place all the ingredients in a bowl and beat until well combined.
3. Pour the dressing over the salad and toss it all to coat well.
4. Serve immediately.

Nutritional Values: Calories 244; Total Fat 16.9 g; Saturated Fat 2.1 g; Cholesterol 0 mg; Sodium 5 mg; Total Carbs 25.2 g; Fiber 5 g; Sugar 18.1 g; Protein 1.8 g

Cauliflower Soup

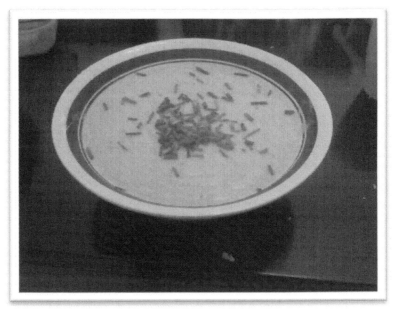

Preparation time: 15 minutes. **Cooking time:** 30 minutes. **Total time:** 45 minutes. **Servings:** 4

Ingredients:

- 2 tbsp olive oil
- 1 yellow onion, chopped
- 2 carrots, peeled and chopped
- 2 celery stalks, chopped
- 2 garlic cloves, minced
- 1 Serrano pepper, chopped finely
- 1 tsp ground turmeric
- 1 tsp ground coriander
- 1 tsp ground cumin

- ¼ tsp red pepper flakes, crushed
- 1 head cauliflower, chopped
- 4 cups homemade vegetable broth
- 1 cup unsweetened coconut milk
- Sea salt and freshly ground black pepper, to taste
- 2 tbsp fresh chives, chopped finely

How to Prepare:

1. In a large soup pan, heat the oil over medium heat and sauté the onion, carrot, and celery for about 4-6 minutes.
2. Add the garlic, Serrano pepper, and spices and sauté for about 1 minute.
3. Add the cauliflower and cook for about 5 minutes, stirring occasionally.
4. Add the broth and coconut milk and bring to a boil over medium-high heat.
5. Reduce the heat to low and simmer for about 15 minutes.
6. Season the soup with the salt and black pepper and remove it from the heat.
7. With an immersion blender, blend the soup until smooth.
8. Serve hot and garnish with chives.

Nutritional Values: Calories 285; Total Fat 23 g; Saturated Fat 14.1 g; Cholesterol 0 mg; Sodium 881 mg; Total Carbs 14.9 g; Fiber 4.8 g; Sugar 7.2 g; Protein 4.5 g

Tomato Soup

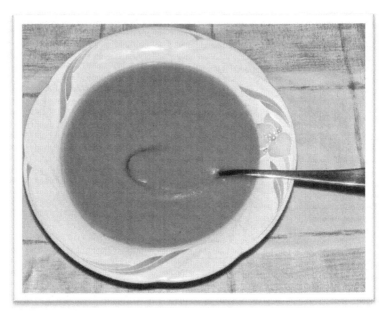

Preparation time: 15 minutes. **Cooking time:** 45 minutes. **Total time:** 1 hour. **Servings:** 4

Ingredients:

- 2 tbsp coconut oil
- 2 carrots, chopped roughly
- 1 large white onion, chopped roughly
- 3 garlic cloves, minced
- 5 large tomatoes, chopped roughly
- 1 tbsp homemade tomato paste
- 3 cups homemade vegetable broth
- ¼ cup fresh basil, chopped
- ¼ cup unsweetened coconut milk
- Sea salt and freshly ground black pepper, to taste

How to Prepare:

1. Melt the coconut oil in a large soup pan over medium heat and cook the carrot and onion for about 10 minutes, stirring frequently.
2. Add the garlic and sauté for about 1-2 minutes.
3. Stir in the tomatoes, tomato paste, basil, broth, salt and black pepper and bring to a boil.
4. Reduce the heat to low and simmer uncovered for about 30 minutes.
5. Stir in the coconut milk and remove from the heat.
6. With an immersion blender, blend the soup until smooth.
7. Serve hot.

Nutritional Values: Calories 197; Total Fat 12 g; Saturated Fat 9.4 g; Cholesterol 0 mg; Sodium 671 mg; Total Carbs 18.4 g; Fiber 4.8 g; Sugar 10.6 g; Protein 7 g

Garlicky Broccoli

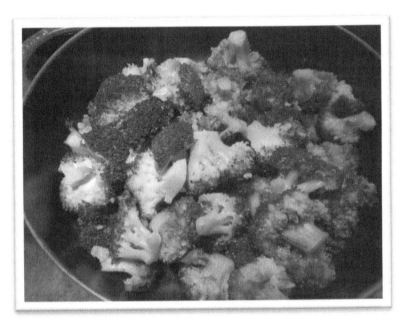

Preparation time: 10 minutes. **Cooking time:** 8 minutes. **Total time:** 18 minutes. **Servings:** 2

Ingredients:

- 1 tbsp extra-virgin olive oil
- 3-4 garlic cloves, minced
- 2 cups broccoli florets
- 2 tbsp tamari

How to Prepare:

1. In a large skillet, heat the oil over medium heat and sauté the garlic for about 1 minute.
2. Add the broccoli and stir fry for about 2 minutes.
3. Stir in the tamari and stir fry for about 4-5 minutes or until desired doneness.
4. Remove from the heat and serve hot.

Nutritional Values: Calories 109; Total Fat 7.3 g; Saturated Fat 1 g; Cholesterol 0 mg; Sodium 1,000 mg; Total Carbs 8.5 g; Fiber 2.6 g; Sugar 1.9 g; Protein 4.7 g

Curried Okra

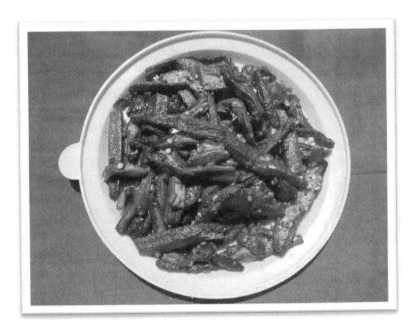

Preparation time: 10 minutes. **Cooking time:** 15 minutes. **Total time:** 25 minutes. **Servings:** 3

Ingredients:

- 1 tbsp olive oil
- ½ tsp cumin seeds
- ¾ lb okra pods, trimmed and cut into 2-inch pieces
- ½ tsp curry powder
- ½ tsp red chili powder
- 1 tsp ground coriander
- Sea salt and freshly ground black pepper, to taste

How to Prepare:

1. In a large skillet, heat the oil over medium heat and sauté the cumin seeds for about 30 seconds.
2. Add the okra and stir fry for about 1-1½ minutes.
3. Reduce the heat to low and cook covered for about 6-8 minutes stirring occasionally.
4. Add the curry powder, red chili, and coriander and stir to combine.
5. Increase the heat to medium and cook uncovered for about 2-3 minutes more.
6. Season with the salt and pepper and remove from the heat.
7. Serve hot.

Nutritional Values: Calories 89; Total Fat 5.1 g; Saturated Fat 0.7 g; Cholesterol 0 mg; Sodium 91 mg; Total Carbs 9 g; Fiber 3.9 g; Sugar 1.7 g; Protein 2.3 g

Mushroom Curry

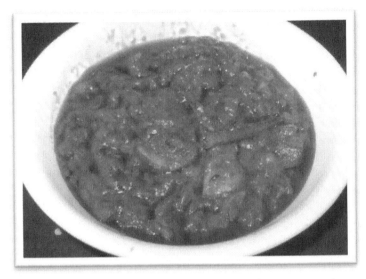

Preparation time: 20 minutes. **Cooking time:** 20 minutes. **Total time:** 40 minutes. **Servings:** 4

Ingredients:

- 2 cup tomatoes, chopped
- 1 green chili, chopped
- 1 tsp fresh ginger, chopped
- 2 tbsp olive oil
- ½ tsp cumin seeds
- ¼ tsp ground coriander
- ¼ tsp ground turmeric
- ¼ tsp red chili powder
- 2 cups fresh shiitake mushrooms, sliced
- 2 cups fresh button mushrooms, sliced
- 1¼ cups water
- ¼ cup unsweetened coconut milk
- Sea salt and freshly ground black pepper, to taste

How to Prepare:

1. In a food processor, add the tomatoes, green chili and ginger and pulse until a smooth paste forms.
2. In a pan, heat the oil over medium heat and sauté the cumin seeds for about 1 minute.
3. Add the spices and sauté for about 1 minute.
4. Add the tomato mixture and cook for about 5 minutes.
5. Stir in the mushrooms, water, and coconut milk and bring to a boil.
6. Cook for about 10-12 minutes, stirring occasionally.
7. Season with the salt and black pepper and remove from the heat.
8. Serve hot.

Nutritional Values: Calories 161; Total Fat 11.2 g; Saturated Fat 4.3 g; Cholesterol 0 mg; Sodium 224 mg; Total Carbs 16.1 g; Fiber 3.5 g; Sugar 6.1 g; Protein 3.5 g

Glazed Brussels Sprouts

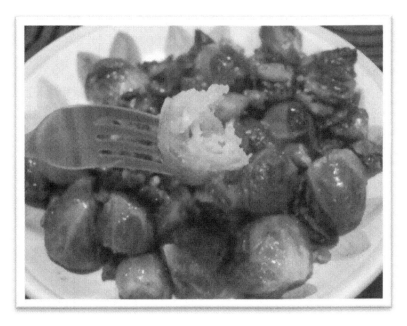

Preparation time: 15 minutes. **Cooking time:** 15 minutes. **Total time:** 30 minutes. **Servings:** 3

Ingredients:

- 3 cups Brussels sprouts, trimmed and halved
- Sea salt, to taste
- 2 tsp coconut oil, melted

For Orange Glaze:

- 1 tsp coconut oil
- 2 small shallots, sliced thinly
- 2 tsp fresh orange zest, grated finely
- ¼ tsp ground ginger

- 2/3 cup fresh orange juice
- 1 tsp sambal oelek (raw chili paste)
- 2 tbsp coconut aminos
- 1 tsp tapioca starch
- Sea salt, to taste

How to Prepare:

1. Preheat the oven to 400 degrees F. Line a roasting pan with parchment paper.
2. In a bowl, add Brussels sprouts, a little salt, and oil and toss to coat well.
3. Transfer the mixture into the prepared roasting pan.
4. Roast for about 10-15 minutes, flipping once halfway through.
5. Meanwhile, prepare the glaze.
6. In a skillet, melt the coconut oil over medium heat and sauté the shallots for about 5 minutes.
7. Add the orange zest and sauté for about 1 minute.
8. Stir in ginger, orange juice, sambal oelek, and coconut aminos and cook for about 5 minutes.
9. Slowly, add the tapioca starch, beating continuously.
10. Cook for about 2-3 minutes more, stirring frequently.
11. Stir in the salt and remove from the heat.
12. Transfer the roasted Brussels sprouts to a serving plate. Top with orange glaze evenly.
13. Serve immediately garnished with scallions.

Nutritional Values: Calories 132; Total Fat 5 g; Saturated Fat 4 g; Cholesterol 0 mg; Sodium 124 mg; Total Carbs 20.6 g; Fiber 4.4 g; Sugar 8.2 g; Protein 3.8 g

Sautéed Mushrooms

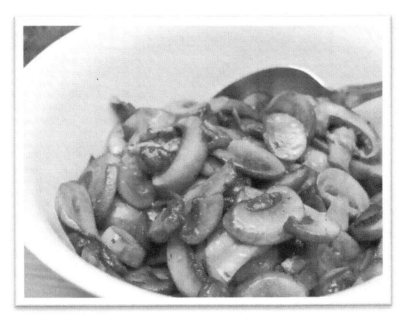

Preparation time: 15 minutes. **Cooking time:** 16 minutes. **Total time:** 31 minutes. **Servings:** 2

Ingredients:

- 2 tbsp olive oil
- ½ tsp cumin seeds, crushed lightly
- 2 medium onions, sliced thinly
- ¾ lb fresh mushrooms, chopped
- Sea salt and freshly ground black pepper, to taste

How to Prepare:

1. In a skillet, heat the oil over medium heat and sauté the cumin seeds for about 1 minute.
2. Add the onion and sauté for about 4-5 minutes.
3. Add the mushrooms and sauté for about 5-7 minutes.
4. Add the salt and black pepper and sauté for about 2-3 minutes.
5. Remove from the heat and serve hot.

Nutritional Values: Calories 202; Total Fat 14.7 g; Saturated Fat 2 g; Cholesterol 0 mg; Sodium 132 mg; Total Carbs 16.1 g; Fiber 4.1 g; Sugar 7.6 g; Protein 66 g

Sweet & Sour Kale

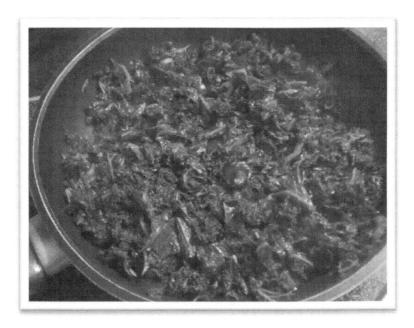

Preparation time: 10 minutes. **Cooking time:** 20 minutes. **Total time:** 30 minutes. **Servings:** 4

Ingredients:

- 1 tbsp extra-virgin olive oil
- 1 lemon, seeded sliced thinly
- 1 onion, chopped
- 3 garlic cloves, minced
- 2 lb fresh kale, tough ribs removed and chopped
- ½ cup scallions, chopped
- 1 tbsp agave nectar
- Sea salt and freshly ground black pepper, to taste

How to Prepare:

1. In a large skillet, heat oil over medium heat and cook the lemon slices for about 5 minutes.
2. With a slotted spoon, remove the lemon slices.
3. In the same skillet, add the onion and garlic and sauté for about 5 minutes.
4. Add the kale, scallions, agave nectar, salt, and black pepper and cook for about 8-10 minutes, stirring occasionally.
5. Remove from the heat and serve hot.

Nutritional Values: Calories 175; Total Fat 3.6 g; Saturated Fat 0.5 g; Cholesterol 0 mg; Sodium 160 mg; Total Carbs 31.9 g; Fiber 4.6 g; Sugar 5.2 g; Protein 7.4 g

Dinner Recipes

Vegetable Soup

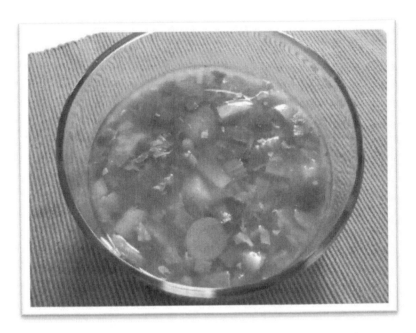

Preparation time: 15 minutes. **Cooking time:** 25 minutes. **Total time:** 40 minutes. **Servings:** 3

Ingredients:

- ½ tbsp olive oil
- 2 tbsp onion, chopped
- 2 tsp garlic, minced
- ½ cup carrots, peeled and chopped
- ½ cup green cabbage, chopped
- 1/3 cup French beans, chopped

- 3 cups homemade vegetable broth
- ½ tbsp fresh lemon juice
- 3 tbsp water
- 2 tbsp arrowroot starch
- Sea salt and freshly ground black pepper, to taste

How to Prepare:

1. Heat the oil in a large, heavy bottomed pan over medium heat and sauté the onion and garlic for about 4-5 minutes.
2. Add the carrots, cabbage, and beans and cook for about 4-5 minutes, stirring frequently.
3. Stir in the broth and bring to a boil.
4. Cook for about 4-5 minutes.
5. Meanwhile, in a small bowl, dissolve the arrowroot starch in water.
6. Slowly, add the arrowroot starch mixture, stirring continuously.
7. Cook for about 7-8 minutes, stirring occasionally.
8. Stir in the lemon juice, salt, and black pepper and remove from the heat.
9. Serve hot.

Nutritional Values: Calories 163; Total Fat 4.2 g; Saturated Fat 0.8 g; Cholesterol 0 mg; Sodium 861 mg; Total Carbs 22.5 g; Fiber 6.3 g; Sugar 2.3 g; Protein 9.2 g

Lentil & Spinach Soup

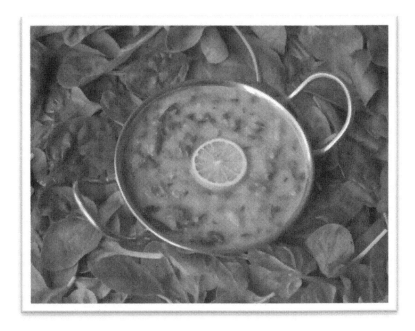

Preparation time: 15 minutes. **Cooking time:** 1¼ hours. **Total time:** 1½ hours. **Servings:** 6

Ingredients:

- 2 tbsp olive oil
- 2 carrots, peeled and chopped
- 2 celery stalks, chopped
- 2 sweet onions, chopped
- 3 garlic cloves, minced
- 1½ cups brown lentils, rinsed
- 2 cups tomatoes, chopped finely
- ¼ tsp dried basil, crushed
- ¼ tsp dried oregano, crushed

60

- ¼ tsp dried thyme, crushed
- 1 tsp ground cumin
- ½ tsp ground coriander
- ½ tsp paprika
- 6 cups vegetable broth
- 3 cups fresh spinach, chopped
- Sea salt and freshly ground black pepper, to taste
- 2 tbsp fresh lemon juice

How to Prepare:

1. In a large soup pan, heat the oil over medium heat and sauté the carrot, celery, and onion for about 5 minutes.
2. Add the garlic and sauté for about 1 minute.
3. Add the lentils and sauté for about 3 minutes.
4. Stir in the tomatoes, herbs, spices, and broth and bring to a boil.
5. Reduce the heat to low and simmer partially covered for about 1 hour or until desired doneness
6. Stir in the spinach, salt, and black pepper and cook for about 4 minutes.
7. Stir in the lemon juice and remove from the heat.
8. Serve hot.

Nutritional Values: Calories 258; Total Fat 1.5 g; Saturated Fat 0.1 g; Cholesterol 0 mg; Sodium 90 mg; Total Carbs 63.6 g; Fiber 13.7 g; Sugar 45.4 g; Protein 5.3 g

Veggie Stew

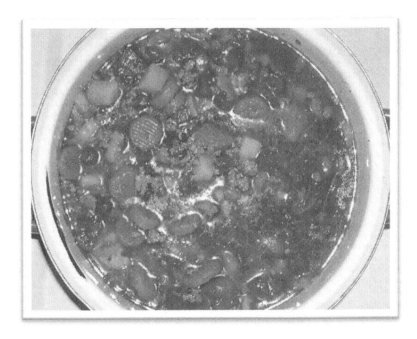

Preparation time: 20 minutes. **Cooking time:** 35 minutes. **Total time:** 55 minutes. **Servings:** 8

Ingredients:

- 2 tbsp coconut oil
- 1 large sweet onion, chopped
- 1 medium parsnip, peeled and chopped
- 3 tbsp homemade tomato paste
- 2 large garlic cloves, minced
- ½ tsp ground cinnamon
- ½ tsp ground ginger
- 1 tsp ground cumin
- ¼ tsp cayenne pepper

- 2 medium carrots, peeled and chopped
- 2 medium purple potatoes, peeled and chopped
- 2 medium sweet potatoes, peeled and chopped
- 4 cups homemade vegetable broth
- 2 cups fresh kale, trimmed and chopped
- 2 tbsp fresh lemon juice
- Sea salt and freshly ground black pepper, to taste

How to Prepare:

1. In a large soup pan, melt the coconut oil over medium-high heat and sauté the onion for about 5 minutes.
2. Add the parsnip and sauté for about 3 minutes.
3. Stir in the tomato paste, garlic, and spices and sauté for about 2 minutes.
4. Stir in carrots, potatoes, sweet potatoes, and broth and bring to a boil.
5. Reduce the heat to medium-low and simmer covered for about 20 minutes.
6. Stir in the kale, lemon juice, salt, and black pepper and simmer for about 5 minutes.
7. Serve hot.

Nutritional Values: Calories 258; Total Fat 1.5 g; Saturated Fat 0.1 g; Cholesterol 0 mg; Sodium 90 mg; Total Carbs 63.6 g; Fiber 13.7 g; Sugar 45.4 g; Protein 5.3 g

Quinoa & Lentil Stew

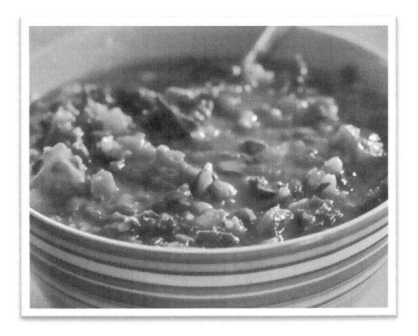

Preparation time: 15 minutes. **Cooking time:** 30 minutes. **Total time:** 45 minutes. **Servings:** 6

Ingredients:

- 1 tbsp coconut oil
- 3 carrots, peeled and chopped
- 3 celery stalks, chopped
- 1 yellow onion, chopped
- 4 garlic cloves, minced
- 4 cups tomatoes, chopped
- 1 cup red lentils, rinsed and drained
- ½ cup dried quinoa, rinsed and drained
- 1½ tsp ground cumin

- 1 tsp red chili powder
- 5 cups vegetable broth
- 2 cups fresh spinach, chopped
- Sea salt and freshly ground black pepper, to taste

How to Prepare:

1. In a large pan, heat the oil over medium heat and sauté the celery, onion, and carrot for about 4-5 minutes.
2. Add the garlic and sauté for about 1 minute.
3. Add the remaining ingredients except the spinach and bring to a boil.
4. Reduce the heat to low and simmer covered for about 20 minutes.
5. Stir in spinach and simmer for about 3-4 minutes.
6. Stir in the salt and black pepper and remove from the heat.
7. Serve hot.

Nutritional Values: Calories 292; Total Fat 6.9 g; Saturated Fat 1.2 g; Cholesterol 0 mg; Sodium 842 mg; Total Carbs 39.1 g; Fiber 17.3 g; Sugar 6.1 g; Protein 19 g

Black Bean Chili

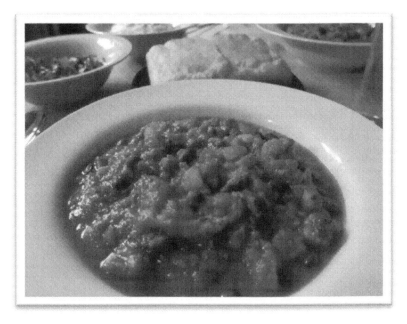

Preparation time: 15 minutes. **Cooking time:** 2 hours 10 minutes. **Total time:** 2 hours 25 minutes. **Servings:** 6

Ingredients:

- 2 tbsp olive oil
- 1 onion, chopped
- 1 small red bell pepper, seeded and chopped
- 1 small green bell pepper, seeded and chopped
- 4 garlic cloves, minced
- 1 tsp ground cumin
- 1 tsp cayenne pepper
- 1 tbsp red chili powder
- 1 medium sweet potato, peeled and chopped

- 3 cups tomatoes, chopped finely
- 4 cups cooked black beans, rinsed and drained
- 2 cups homemade vegetable broth
- Sea salt and freshly ground black pepper, to taste

How to Prepare:

1. In a large pan, heat the oil over medium-high heat and sauté the onion and bell peppers for about 3-4 minutes.
2. Add the garlic and spices and sauté for about 1 minute.
3. Add the sweet potato and cook for about 4-5 minutes.
4. Add the remaining ingredients and bring to a boil.
5. Reduce the heat to medium-low and simmer covered for about 1½-2 hours.
6. Season with the salt and black pepper and remove from the heat.
7. Serve hot.

Nutritional Values: Calories 275; Total Fat 7.2 g; Saturated Fat 0.9 g; Cholesterol 0 mg; Sodium 613 mg; Total Carbs 40.8 g; Fiber 11.2 g; Sugar 12 g; Protein 13.1 g

Kidney Bean Curry

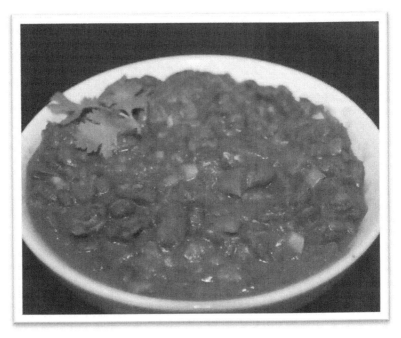

Preparation time: 15 minutes. **Cooking time:** 25 minutes. **Total time:** 40 minutes. **Servings:** 6

Ingredients:

- ¼ cup extra-virgin olive oil
- 1 medium onion, chopped finely
- 2 garlic cloves, minced
- 2 tbsp fresh ginger, minced
- 1 cup homemade tomato puree
- 1 tsp ground coriander
- 1 tsp ground cumin
- ½ tsp ground turmeric

- ¼ tsp cayenne pepper
- Sea salt and freshly ground black pepper, to taste
- 2 large plum tomatoes, chopped finely
- 3 cups boiled red kidney beans
- 2 cups water
- ½ cup fresh parsley, chopped

How to Prepare:

1. In a large soup pan, heat the oil over medium heat and sauté the onion, garlic, and ginger for about 4-5 minutes.
2. Stir in the tomato puree and spices and cook for about 5 minutes.
3. Stir in the tomatoes, kidney beans, and water and bring to a boil over high heat.
4. Reduce the heat to medium and simmer for about 10-15 minutes or until desired thickness.
5. Serve hot and garnish with parsley.

Nutritional Values: Calories 228; Total Fat 9.9 g; Saturated Fat 1.3 g; Cholesterol 0 mg; Sodium 341 mg; Total Carbs 28.1 g; Fiber 8.4 g; Sugar 5.5 g; Protein 8.9 g

Green Bean Casserole

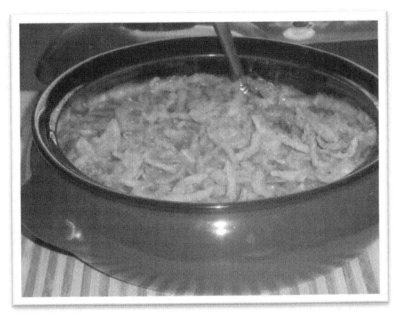

Preparation time: 20 minutes. **Cooking time:** 20 minutes. **Total time:** 40 minutes. **Servings:** 6

Ingredients:

For Onion Slices:

- ½ cup yellow onion, sliced very thinly
- ¼ cup almond flour
- 1/8 tsp garlic powder
- Sea salt and freshly ground black pepper, to taste

For Casserole:

- 1 lb fresh green beans, trimmed
- 1 tbsp olive oil
- 8 oz fresh cremini mushrooms, sliced
- ½ cup yellow onion, sliced thinly
- 1/8 tsp garlic powder
- Sea salt and freshly ground black pepper, to taste

- 1 tsp fresh thyme, chopped
- ½ cup homemade vegetable broth
- ½ cup coconut cream

How to Prepare:

1. Preheat the oven to 350 degrees F.
2. For onion slices, place all the ingredients in a bowl and toss them to coat the onion well.
3. Arrange the onion slices onto a large baking sheet in a single layer and set it aside.
4. In a pan of salted boiling water, add the green beans and cook for about 5 minutes.
5. Drain the green beans and transfer them into a bowl of ice water.
6. Again, drain well and transfer them again into a large bowl. Set them aside.
7. In a large skillet, heat oil over medium-high heat and sauté the mushrooms, onion, garlic powder, salt, and black pepper for about 2-3 minutes.
8. Stir in the thyme and broth and cook for about 3-5 minutes or until all the liquid is absorbed.
9. Remove from the heat and transfer the mushroom mixture into the bowl with the green beans.
10. Add the coconut cream and stir to combine well.
11. Transfer the mixture into a 10-inch casserole dish.
12. Place the casserole dish and baking sheet of onion slices into the oven.
13. Bake for about 15-17 minutes.
14. Remove the baking dish and sheet from the oven and let it cool for about 5 minutes before serving.
15. Top the casserole with the crispy onion slices evenly.
16. Cut into 6 equal-sized portions and serve.

Nutritional Values: Calories 138; Total Fat 9.7 g; Saturated Fat 4.8 g; Cholesterol 0 mg; Sodium 101 mg; Total Carbs 11.1 g; Fiber 4.2 g; Sugar 3.4 g; Protein 4.4 g

Vegetarian Pie

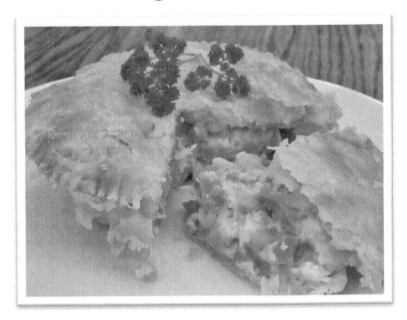

Preparation time: 20 minutes. **Cooking time:** 1 hour 20 minutes. **Total time:** 1 hour 40 minute. **Servings:** 8

Ingredients:

For Topping:

- 5 cups water
- 1¼ cups yellow cornmeal

For Filing:

- 1 tbsp extra-virgin olive oil
- 1 large onion, chopped
- 1 medium red bell pepper, seeded and chopped
- 2 garlic cloves, minced
- 1 tsp dried oregano, crushed
- 2 tsp chili powder

- 2 cups fresh tomatoes, chopped
- 2½ cups cooked pinto beans
- 2 cups boiled corn kernels

How to Prepare:

1. Preheat the oven to 375 degrees F. Lightly grease a shallow baking dish.
2. In a pan, add the water over medium-high heat and bring to a boil.
3. Slowly, add the cornmeal, stirring continuously.
4. Reduce the heat to low and cook covered for about 20 minutes, stirring occasionally.
5. Meanwhile, prepare the filling. In a large skillet, heat the oil over medium heat and sauté the onion and bell pepper for about 3-4 minutes.
6. Add the garlic, oregano, and spices and sauté for about 1 minute
7. Add the remaining ingredients and stir to combine.
8. Reduce the heat to low and simmer for about 10-15 minutes, stirring occasionally.
9. Remove from the heat.
10. Place half of the cooked cornmeal into the prepared baking dish evenly.
11. Place the filling mixture over the cornmeal evenly.
12. Place the remaining cornmeal over the filling mixture evenly.
13. Bake for 45-50 minutes or until the top becomes golden brown.
14. Remove the pie from the oven and set it aside for about 5 minutes before serving.

Nutritional Values: Calories 350; Total Fat 3.9 g; Saturated Fat 0.6 g; Cholesterol 0 mg; Sodium 34 mg; Total Carbs 65 g; Fiber 13.3 g; Sugar 5.4 g; Protein 16.6 g

Rice & Lentil Loaf

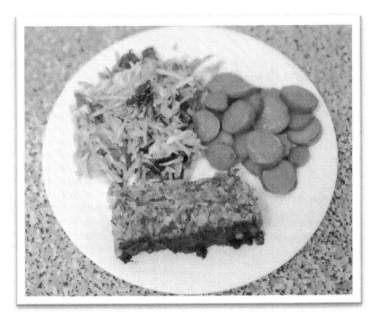

Preparation time: 20 minutes. **Cooking time:** 1 hour 50 minutes. **Total time:** 2 hours 10 minutes. **Servings:** 8

Ingredients:

- 1¾ cups plus 2 tbsp filtered water, divided
- ½ cup wild rice
- ½ cup brown lentils; Pinch of sea salt
- ½ tsp no-sodium Italian seasoning
- 1 medium yellow onion, chopped
- 1 celery stalk, chopped
- 6 cremini mushrooms, chopped
- 4 garlic cloves, minced; ¾ cup rolled oats
- ½ cup pecans, chopped finely
- ¾ cup homemade tomato sauce
- ½ tsp red pepper flakes, crushed
- 1 tsp fresh rosemary, minced; 2 tsp fresh thyme, minced

How to Prepare:

1. In a pan, add 1¾ cups of water, rice, lentils, salt, and Italian seasoning and bring them to a boil over medium-high heat.
2. Reduce the heat to low and simmer covered for about 45 minutes.
3. Remove from the heat and set it aside still covered for at least 10 minutes.
4. Preheat the oven to 350 degrees F. Line a 9x5-inch loaf pan with parchment paper.
5. In a skillet, heat the remaining water over medium heat and sauté the onion, celery, mushrooms, and garlic for about 4-5 minutes.
6. Remove from the heat and let it cool slightly.
7. In a large mixing bowl, add the oats, pecans, tomato sauce, and fresh herbs and mix until well combined.
8. Combine the rice mixture and vegetable mixture with the oat mixture and mix well.
9. In a blender, add the mixture and pulse until a chunky mixture forms.
10. Transfer the mixture into the prepared loaf pan evenly.
11. With a piece of foil, cover the loaf pan and bake it for about 40 minutes.
12. Uncover and bake for about 15-20 minutes more or until the top becomes golden brown.
13. Remove it from the oven and set it aside for about 5-10 minutes before slicing.
14. Cut into desired sized slices and serve.

Nutritional Values: Calories 179; Total Fat 6.6 g; Saturated Fat 0.7 g; Cholesterol 0 mg; Sodium 157 mg; Total Carbs 24.6 g; Fiber 6.8 g; Sugar 2.6 g; Protein 7.1 g

Asparagus Risotto

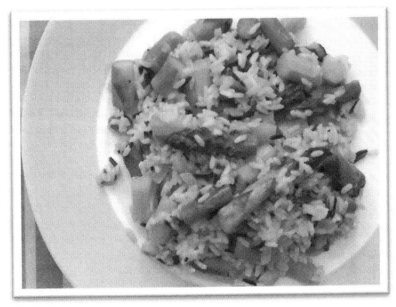

Preparation time: 15 minutes. **Cooking time:** 45 minutes. **Total time:** 1 hour. **Servings:** 4

Ingredients:

- 15-20 fresh asparagus spears, trimmed and cut into 1½-inch pieces
- 2 tbsp olive oil
- 1 cup yellow onion, chopped
- 1 garlic clove, minced
- 1 cup Arborio rice
- 1 tbsp fresh lemon zest, grated finely
- 2 tbsp fresh lemon juice
- 5½ cups hot vegetable broth
- 1 tbsp fresh parsley, chopped
- ¼ cup nutritional yeast
- Sea salt and freshly ground black pepper, to taste

How to Prepare:

1. Boil water in a medium pan then add asparagus and cook for about 3 minutes.
2. Drain the asparagus and rinse under cold running water.
3. Drain well and set aside.
4. In a large pan, heat oil over medium heat and sauté the onion for about 5 minutes.
5. Add the garlic and sauté for about 1 minute.
6. Add the rice and stir fry for about 2 minutes.
7. Add the lemon zest, lemon juice, and ½ cup of broth and cook for about 3 minutes or until all the liquid is absorbed, stirring gently.
8. Add 1 cup of broth and cook until all the broth is absorbed, stirring occasionally.
9. Repeat this process by adding ¾ cup of broth at a time until all the broth is absorbed, stirring occasionally. (This procedure will take about 20-30 minutes.)
10. Stir in the cooked asparagus and remaining ingredients and cook for about 4 minutes.
11. Serve hot.

Nutritional Values: Calories 353; Total Fat 9.9 g; Saturated Fat 1.8 g; Cholesterol 0 mg; Sodium 1,100 mg; Total Carbs 50.5 g; Fiber 6.5 g; Sugar 4.1 g; Protein 16.9 g

Dessert Recipes

Baked Apples

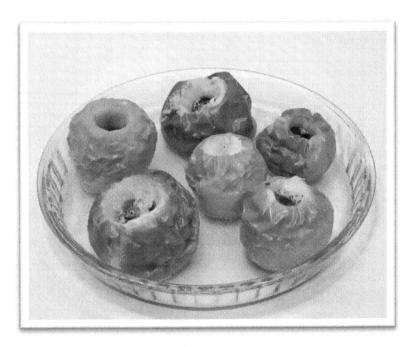

Preparation time: 15 minutes. **Cooking time:** 18 minutes. **Total time:** 33 minutes. **Servings:** 4

Ingredients:

- 4 apples, cored
- ¼ cup coconut oil, softened
- 4 tsp ground cinnamon
- 1/8 tsp ground ginger
- 1/8 tsp ground nutmeg

How to Prepare:

1. Preheat the oven to 350 degrees F.
2. Fill each apple with 1 tablespoon of coconut oil.
3. Sprinkle each with spices evenly.
4. Arrange the apples on a baking sheet.
5. Bake for about 12-18 minutes.

Nutritional Values: Calories 240; Total Fat 14.1 g; Saturated Fat 11.8 g; Cholesterol 0 mg; Sodium 2 mg; Total Carbs 32.7 g; Fiber 6.6 g; Sugar 23.3 g; Protein 0.7 g

Berries Granita

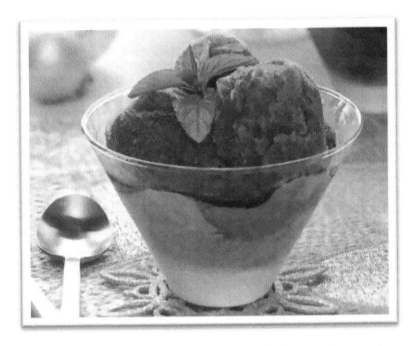

Preparation time: 15 minutes. **Total time:** About 3 hours.
Servings: 4

Ingredients:

- ½ cup fresh strawberries, hulled and sliced
- ½ cup fresh raspberries
- ½ cup fresh blueberries
- ½ cup fresh blackberries
- 1 tbsp pure maple syrup
- 1 tbsp fresh lemon juice
- 1 cup ice cubes, crushed
- 1 tsp fresh mint leaves

How to Prepare:

1. In a high-speed blender, add the berries, maple syrup, lemon juice, and ice cubes and pulse on high speed until smooth.
2. Transfer the berries mixture into an 8x8-inch baking dish evenly and freeze for at least 30 minutes.
3. Remove from the freezer and stir the granita completely using a fork.
4. Return it to the freezer and freeze it for about 2-3 hours. Scrape it every 30 minutes with a fork.
5. Place the granita into serving glasses and serve immediately garnished with mint leaves.

Nutritional Values: Calories 46; Total Fat 0.3 g; Saturated Fat 0 g; Cholesterol 0 mg; Sodium 4 mg; Total Carbs 11.1 g; Fiber 2.8 g; Sugar 7.3 g; Protein 0.7 g

Pumpkin Ice Cream

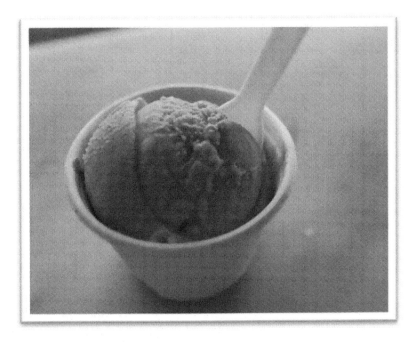

Preparation time: 15 minutes. **Total time:** 2¼ hours. **Servings:** 6

Note: This recipe calls for the use of an ice cream machine.

Ingredients:

- 15 oz homemade pumpkin puree
- ½ cup dates, pitted and chopped
- 2 (14-oz) cans unsweetened coconut milk
- ½ tsp organic vanilla extract
- 1½ tsp pumpkin pie spice
- ½ tsp ground cinnamon
- Pinch of sea salt

How to Prepare:

1. In a high speed blender, add all the ingredients and pulse until smooth.
2. Transfer into an airtight container and freeze for about 1-2 hours.
3. Now, transfer the mixture into an ice cream maker and process it according to the manufacturer's directions.
4. Return the ice cream to the airtight container and freeze for about 1-2 hours before serving.

Nutritional Values: Calories 293; Total Fat 22.5 g; Saturated Fat 20.1 g; Cholesterol 0 mg; Sodium 99 mg; Total Carbs 24.8 g; Fiber 3.6 g; Sugar 14.1 g; Protein 2.3 g

Lemon Sorbet

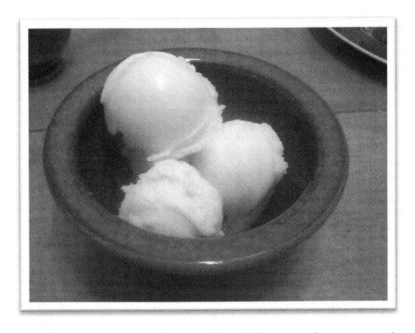

Preparation time: 10 minutes. **Total time:** 2 hours 10 minutes.
Servings: 4

Note: This recipe calls for the use of an ice cream maker.

Ingredients:

- 2 tbsp fresh lemon zest, grated
- ½ cup pure maple syrup
- 2 cups water
- 1½ cups fresh lemon juice

How to Prepare:

1. Freeze ice cream maker tub for about 24 hours before making this sorbet.
2. Add all of the ingredients except the lemon juice in a pan and simmer them over medium heat for about 1 minute or until the sugar dissolves, stirring continuously.
3. Remove the pan from the heat and stir in the lemon juice.
4. Transfer this into an airtight container and refrigerate for about 2 hours.
5. Now, transfer the mixture into an ice cream maker and process it according to the manufacturer's directions.
6. Return the ice cream to the airtight container and freeze for about 2 hours.

Nutritional Values: Calories 127; Total Fat 0.8 g; Saturated Fat 0.7 g; Cholesterol 0 mg; Sodium 26 mg; Total Carbs 29 g; Fiber 0.6 g; Sugar 25.5 g; Protein 0.8 g

Avocado Pudding

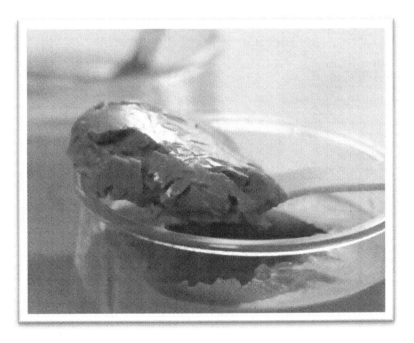

Preparation time: 15 minutes. **Total time:** 3¼ hours. **Servings:** 4

Ingredients:

- 2 cups bananas, peeled and chopped
- 2 ripe avocados, peeled, pitted, and chopped
- 1 tsp fresh lime zest, grated finely
- 1 tsp fresh lemon zest, grated finely
- ½ cup fresh lime juice
- ½ cup fresh lemon juice
- 1/3 cup agave nectar

How to Prepare:

1. In a blender, add all the ingredients and pulse until smooth.
2. Transfer the mousse into 4 serving glasses and refrigerate to chill for about 3 hours before serving.

Nutritional Values: Calories 462; Total Fat 20.1 g; Saturated Fat 4.4 g; Cholesterol 0 mg; Sodium 13 mg; Total Carbs 48.2 g; Fiber 10.2 g; Sugar 30.4 g; Protein 3 g

Chocolate Mousse

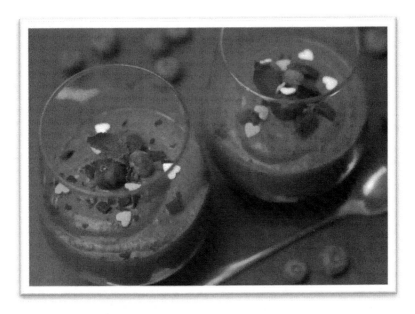

Preparation time: 10 minutes. **Total time:** 10 minutes.

Servings: 4

Ingredients:

- ½ cup unsweetened almond milk
- 1 cup cooked black beans
- 4 Medjool dates, pitted and chopped
- ½ cup pecans, chopped
- 2 tbsp non-alkalized cocoa powder
- 1 tsp organic vanilla extract
- 4 tbsp fresh blueberries

How to Prepare:

1. In a food processor, add all the ingredients and pulse until smooth and creamy.
2. Transfer the mixture into serving bowls and refrigerate to chill before serving.
3. Garnish with blueberries and serve.

Nutritional Values: Calories 357; Total Fat 13 g; Saturated Fat 1.7 g; Cholesterol 0 mg; Sodium 26 mg; Total Carbs 52.1 g; Fiber 11.9 g; Sugar 16.7 g; Protein 13.4 g

Blueberry Crumble

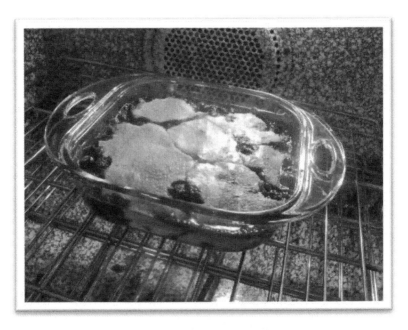

Preparation time: 15 minutes. **Cooking time:** 40 minutes. **Total time:** 55 minutes. **Servings:** 4

Ingredients:

- ¼ cup coconut flour
- ¼ cup arrowroot flour
- ¾ tsp baking soda
- ¼ cup ripe banana, peeled and mashed
- 2 tbsp coconut oil, melted
- 3 tbsp filtered water
- ½ tbsp fresh lemon juice
- 1½ cups fresh blueberries

How to Prepare:

1. Preheat the oven to 300 degrees F. Lightly grease an 8x8-inch baking dish.
2. In a large bowl, add all the ingredients except the blueberries and mix until well combined.
3. In the bottom of the prepared baking dish, place the blueberries and top them with the flour mixture evenly.
4. Bake for about 40 minutes or until the top becomes golden brown.
5. Serve warm.

Nutritional Values: Calories 107; Total Fat 7.2 g; Saturated Fat 6 g; Cholesterol 0 mg; Sodium 240 mg; Total Carbs 11.6 g; Fiber 2 g; Sugar 6.7 g; Protein 1 g

Apple Crisp

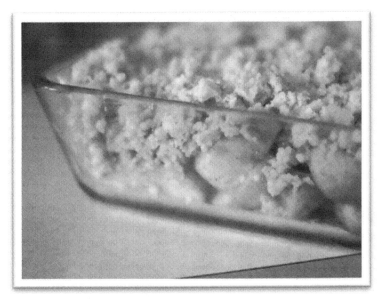

Preparation time: 15 minutes. **Cooking time:** 20 minutes. **Total time:** 35 minutes. **Servings:** 8

Ingredients:

For Filling:
- 2 large apples, peeled, cored, and chopped
- 2 tbsp water
- 2 tbsp fresh apple juice
- ¼ tsp ground cinnamon

For Topping:
- ½ cup quick rolled oats
- ¼ cup unsweetened coconut flakes
- 2 tbsp pecans, chopped
- ½ tsp ground cinnamon
- ¼ cup water

How to Prepare:

1. Preheat the oven to 300F. Lightly grease a baking dish.
2. To make the filling add all of the ingredients in a large bowl and gently mix. Set this aside.
3. Make the topping by adding all of the ingredients to another bowl and mix well.
4. Place the filling mixture into the prepared baking dish then spread the topping over the filling mixture evenly.
5. Bake for about 20 minutes or until the top becomes golden brown.
6. Serve warm.

Nutritional Values: Calories 100; Total Fat 2.7 g; Saturated Fat 0.8 g; Cholesterol 0 mg; Sodium 3 mg; Total Carbs 19.1 g; Fiber 2.6 g; Sugar 11.9 g; Protein 1.2 g

Coconut Macaroons

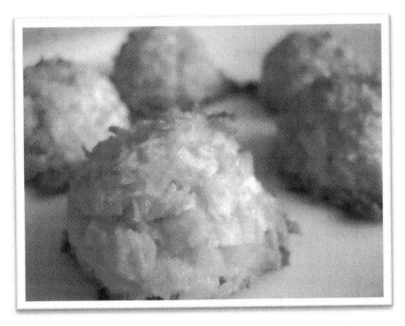

Preparation time: 15 minutes. **Cooking time:** 10 minutes. **Total time:** 25 minutes. **Servings:** 12

Ingredients:

- 1½ cups unsweetened coconut, shredded
- 1 tbsp coconut flour
- 1/8 tsp sea salt
- ¼ cup pure maple syrup
- 2 tbsp coconut oil, melted
- 1 tbsp organic vanilla extract

How to Prepare:

1. Preheat the oven to 350 degrees F. Line a large cookie sheet with parchment paper.
2. In a food processor, add all the ingredients and pulse until well combined.
3. Divide the mixture up into tablespoon-size portions and place them onto the prepared cookie sheet in a single layer.
4. Bake for about 7-10 minutes or until golden brown.
5. Remove from the oven and let them cool for about 1 hour before serving.

Nutritional Values: Calories 78; Total Fat 5.7 g; Saturated Fat 5g; Cholesterol 0 mg; Sodium 22 mg; Total Carbs 6.5 g; Fiber 1.2 g; Sugar 4.7 g; Protein 0.4 g

Chickpea Fudge

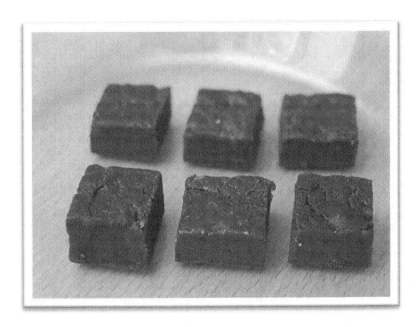

Preparation time: 15 minutes. **Total time:** 15 minutes.

Servings: 12

Ingredients:

- 2 cups cooked chickpeas
- 8 Medjool dates, pitted and chopped
- ½ cup almond butter
- ½ cup unsweetened almond milk
- 1 tsp organic vanilla extract
- 2 tbsp cacao powder

How to Prepare:

1. Line a large baking dish with parchment paper.
2. In a food processor, add all ingredients except the cacao powder and pulse until well combined.
3. Transfer the mixture into a large bowl and stir in the cacao powder.
4. Transfer the mixture onto the prepared baking dish evenly and smooth the surface with the back of a spatula.
5. Refrigerate for about 2 hours or until set completely.
6. Cut into desired sized squares and serve.

Nutritional Values: Calories 172; Total Fat 2.8 g; Saturated Fat 0.3 g; Cholesterol 0 mg; Sodium 16 mg; Total Carbs 32 g; Fiber 7.4 g; Sugar 13 g; Protein 7.1 g

Smoothie Recipes

Oats & Orange Smoothie

Preparation time: 10 minutes. **Total time:** 10 minutes.
Servings: 4

Ingredients:

- 2/3 cups rolled oats
- 2 oranges, peeled, seeded, and sectioned
- 2 large bananas, peeled and sliced
- 2 cups unsweetened almond milk
- 1 cup ice cubes, crushed

How to Prepare:

1. Place all the ingredients in a high-speed blender and pulse until creamy.
2. Pour the smoothie into four glasses and serve immediately.

Nutritional Values: Calories 175; Total Fat 3 g; Saturated Fat 0.4 g; Cholesterol 0 mg; Sodium 93 mg; Total Carbs 36.6 g; Fiber 5.9 g; Sugar 11.7 g; Protein 5.9 g

Spiced Banana Smoothie

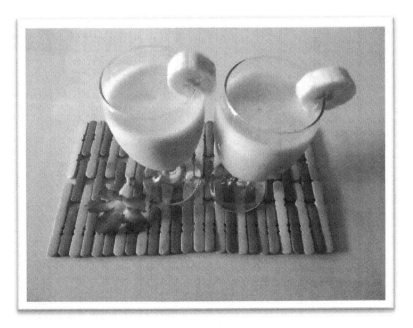

Preparation time: 5 minutes. **Total time:** 5 minutes. **Servings:** 2

Ingredients:

- 2 medium frozen bananas, peeled and sliced
- 1 tsp organic vanilla extract
- ¼ tsp ground cinnamon
- Pinch of ground nutmeg
- Pinch of ground cloves
- 1½ cups unsweetened almond milk

How to Prepare:

1. Place all the ingredients in a high-speed blender and pulse until creamy.
2. Pour the smoothie into two glasses and serve immediately.

Nutritional Values: Calories 143; Total Fat 2.1 g; Saturated Fat 0.4 g; Cholesterol 0 mg; Sodium 137 mg; Total Carbs 29.1 g; Fiber 4 g; Sugar 14.8 g; Protein 2.1 g

Blueberry Smoothie

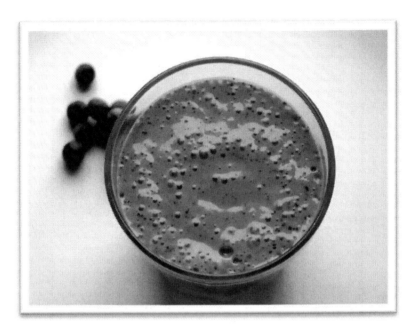

Preparation time: 5 minutes. **Total time:** 5 minutes. **Servings:** 2

Ingredients:

- 2 cups frozen blueberries
- 1 small banana, peeled and sliced
- 1½ cups unsweetened almond milk
- ¼ cup ice cubes

How to Prepare:

1. Place all the ingredients in a high-speed blender and pulse until creamy.
2. Pour the smoothie into two glasses and serve immediately.

Nutritional Values: Calories 158; Total Fat 3.3 g; Saturated Fat 0.3 g; Cholesterol 0 mg; Sodium 137 mg; Total Carbs 34 g; Fiber 5.6 g; Sugar 20 g; Protein 2.2 g

Raspberry & Tofu Smoothie

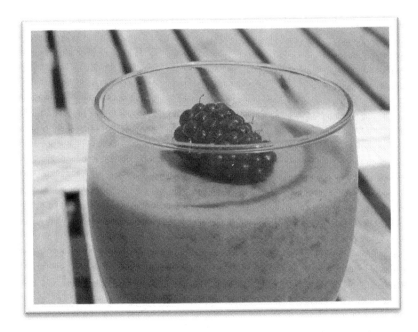

Preparation time: 10 minutes. **Total time:** 10 minutes.

Servings: 2

Ingredients:

- 8 oz firm silken tofu, pressed and drained
- 1 cup frozen raspberries
- ¼ tsp coconut extract
- 4-6 drops liquid stevia
- 1 cup coconut cream
- ½ cup ice cubes, crushed

How to Prepare:

1. Place all the ingredients in a high-speed blender and pulse until creamy.
2. Pour the smoothie into two glasses and serve immediately.

Nutritional Values: Calories 328; Total Fat 15.4 g; Saturated Fat 9.7 g; Cholesterol 0 mg; Sodium 32 mg; Total Carbs 39.4 g; Fiber 6.5 g; Sugar 28 g; Protein 11.4g

Papaya Smoothie

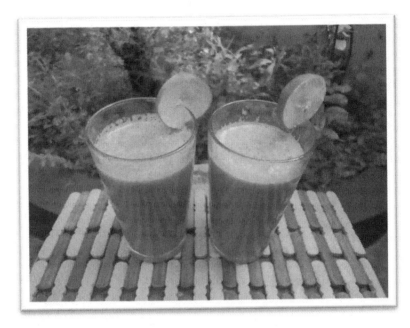

Preparation time: 10 minutes. **Total time:** 10 minutes.

Servings: 2

Ingredients:

- 1 large banana, peeled and sliced
- ½ medium papaya, peeled and chopped roughly
- 1½ cups unsweetened almond milk
- 2 tbsp agave syrup
- 1 tbsp fresh lime juice
- ¼ tsp ground turmeric
- ½ cup ice cubes, crushed

How to Prepare:

1. Place all the ingredients in a high-speed blender and pulse until creamy.
2. Pour the smoothie into two glasses and serve immediately.

Nutritional Values: Calories 190; Total Fat 3.1 g; Saturated Fat 0.4 g; Cholesterol 0 mg; Sodium 157 mg; Total Carbs 42.6 g; Fiber 3.9 g; Sugar 14.5 g; Protein 1.9 g

Peach Smoothie

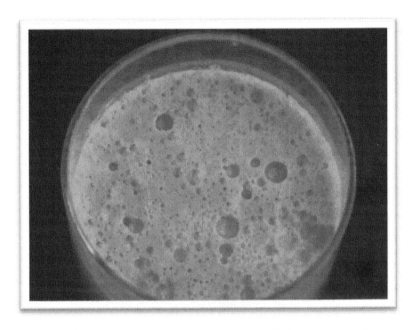

Preparation time: 10 minutes. **Total time:** 10 minutes.

Servings: 2

Ingredients:

- 1 large peach, peeled, pitted, and chopped
- 1 medium frozen banana, peeled and sliced
- 2 oz aloe vera
- ½ tsp fresh ginger, peeled and chopped
- 2 tbsp flax seeds
- ½ tsp organic vanilla extract
- 1¾ cups unsweetened almond milk

How to Prepare:

1. Add all the ingredients in a high-speed blender and pulse until smooth.
2. Pour the smoothie into two glasses and serve immediately.

Nutritional Values: Calories 162; Total Fat 5.7 g; Saturated Fat 0.6 g; Cholesterol 0 mg; Sodium 160 mg; Total Carbs 25.7g; Fiber 5.5 g; Sugar 14.5 g; Protein 3.6 g

Strawberry & Beet Smoothie

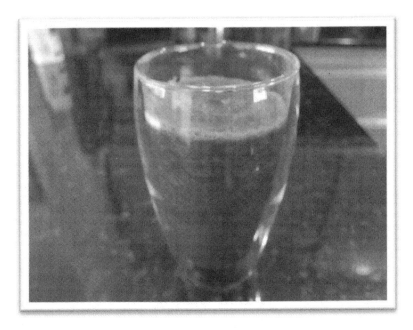

Preparation time: 10 minutes. **Total time:** 10 minutes.

Servings: 2

Ingredients:

- 2 cups frozen strawberries, pitted and chopped
- 2/3 cup frozen beets, chopped
- 1 tsp fresh ginger, peeled and grated
- 1 tsp fresh turmeric, peeled and grated
- ½ cup fresh orange juice
- 1 cup unsweetened almond milk

How to Prepare:

1. Add all the ingredients in a high-speed blender and pulse until smooth.
2. Pour the smoothie into two glasses and serve immediately.

Nutritional Values: Calories 130; Total Fat 2.1 g; Saturated Fat 0.2 g; Cholesterol 0 mg; Sodium 135 mg; Total Carbs 27.5 g; Fiber 5.1 g; Sugar 18.7 g; Protein 2 g

Grape & Swiss Chard Smoothie

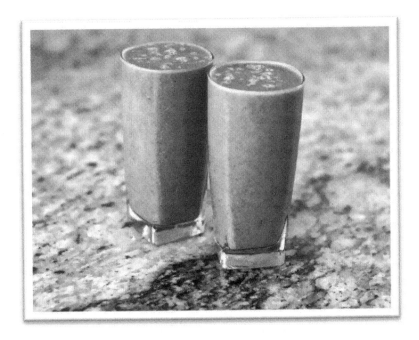

Preparation time: 10 minutes. **Total time:** 10 minutes.

Servings: 2

Ingredients:

- 2 cups seedless green grapes
- 2 cups fresh Swiss chard, trimmed and chopped
- 2 tbsp agave nectar
- 1 tsp fresh lemon juice
- 1½ cups alkaline water
- ¼ cup ice cubes, crushed

How to Prepare:

1. Add all the ingredients in a high-speed blender and pulse until smooth.
2. Pour the smoothie into two glasses and serve immediately.

Nutritional Values: Calories 128; Total Fat 1.1 g; Saturated Fat 0 g; Cholesterol 0 mg; Sodium 78 mg; Total Carbs 33.4 g; Fiber 2.6 g; Sugar 30.5 g; Protein 1.7g;

Kale Smoothie

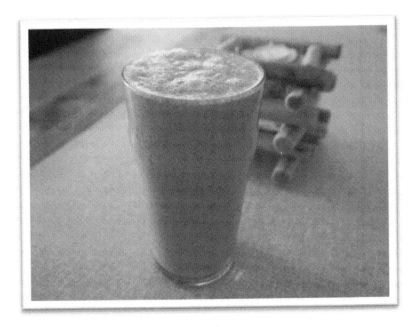

Preparation time: 10 minutes. **Total time:** 10 minutes.

Servings: 2

Ingredients:

- 1 cup fresh kale, tough ribs removed and chopped
- 1-2 celery stalks, chopped
- ½ avocado, peeled, pitted, and chopped
- ½-1 ginger root, chopped
- ½ turmeric root, chopped
- 1½ cups unsweetened coconut milk
- ¼ cup ice cubes, crushed

How to Prepare:

1. Add all the ingredients in a high-speed blender and pulse until smooth.
2. Pour the smoothie into two glasses and serve immediately.

Nutritional Values: Calories 158; Total Fat 12.9 g; Saturated Fat 5.1 g; Cholesterol 0 mg; Sodium 26 mg; Total Carbs 10.3 g; Fiber 4.9 g; Sugar 0.4 g; Protein 2.1 g

Green Veggie Smoothie

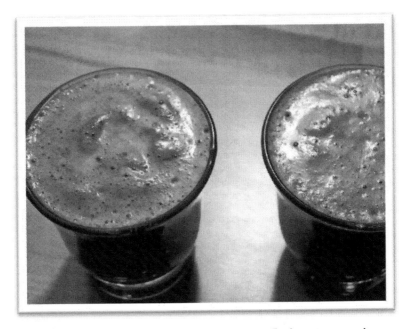

Preparation time: 10 minutes. **Total time:** 10 minutes.

Servings: 2

Ingredients:

- ½ small cucumber, peeled and chopped roughly
- 1 cup fresh dandelion greens, chopped
- 1 celery stalk, chopped
- ¼ tsp fresh ginger, chopped
- 8-10 drops liquid stevia
- ½ tbsp fresh lime juice
- 1½ cups alkaline water
- ¼ cup ice cubes, crushed

How to Prepare:

1. Add all the ingredients in a high-speed blender and pulse until smooth.
2. Pour the smoothie into two glasses and serve immediately.

Nutritional Values: Calories 26; Total Fat 0.3 g; Saturated Fat 0.1 g; Cholesterol 0 mg; Sodium 30 mg; Total Carbs 5.7 g; Fiber 1.5 g; Sugar 1.6 g; Protein 1.3 g

Snack Recipes

Chocolate Milkshake

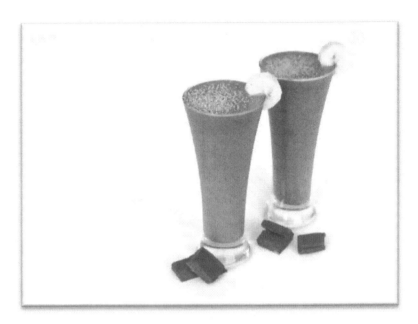

Preparation time: 10 minutes. **Total time:** 10 minutes.
Servings: 2

Ingredients:

- 2 large frozen bananas, peeled
- 1 tbsp almond butter
- 1 tbsp cacao powder
- ¼ tsp organic vanilla extract
- 1½ cups unsweetened almond milk

How to Prepare:

1. Add all the ingredients in a high-speed blender and pulse until smooth.
2. Pour the milkshake into two glasses and serve immediately.

Nutritional Values: Calories 208; Total Fat 8.1 g; Saturated Fat 1 g; Cholesterol 0 mg; Sodium 137 mg; Total Carbs 35.4 g; Fiber 5.8 g; Sugar 17.1 g; Protein 4.4 g

Strawberry Gazpacho

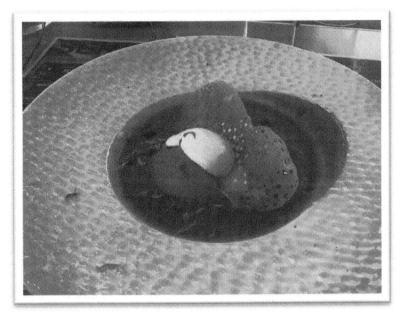

Preparation time: 15 minutes. **Total time:** 15 minutes.

Servings: 4

Ingredients:

- 1½ lbs fresh strawberries, hulled and sliced plus more for garnishing
- ½ cup red bell pepper, seeded and chopped
- 1 small cucumber, peeled, seeded, and chopped
- ¼ cup onion, chopped
- ¼ cup fresh basil leaves
- 1 small garlic clove, chopped
- ¼ small jalapeño pepper, seeded and chopped
- 1 tbsp olive oil
- 3 tbsp balsamic vinegar

How to Prepare:

1. In a high-seed blender, add 1½ pounds of the strawberries and the remaining ingredients and pulse until well combined and smooth.
2. Transfer the gazpacho into a large serving bowl.
3. Cover the bowl and refrigerate to chill completely before serving.
4. Serve chilled garnished with extra strawberry slices.

Nutritional Values: Calories 107; Total Fat 4.2 g; Saturated Fat 0.5 g; Cholesterol 0 mg; Sodium 5 mg; Total Carbs 17.8 g; Fiber 4.2 g; Sugar 10.8 g; Protein 1.1 g

Tomato Salsa

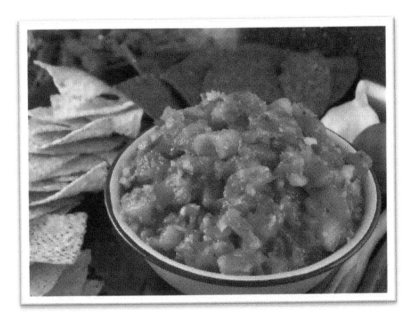

Preparation time: 15 minutes. **Total time:** 15 minutes.
Servings: 4

Ingredients:

- 3 large tomatoes, chopped
- 1 small red onion, chopped
- ¼ cup fresh cilantro leaves, chopped
- 1 jalapeño pepper, seeded and chopped finely
- 1 small garlic clove, minced finely
- 2 tbsp fresh lime juice
- 1 tbsp extra-virgin olive oil
- Sea salt and freshly ground black pepper, to taste

How to Prepare:

1. In a large bowl, add all the ingredients and gently toss to coat well.
2. Serve immediately.

Nutritional Values: Calories 64; Total Fat 3.8 g; Saturated Fat 0.5 g; Cholesterol 0 mg; Sodium 66 mg; Total Carbs 7.5 g; Fiber 2.2 g; Sugar 4.5 g; Protein 15 g

Avocado Guacamole

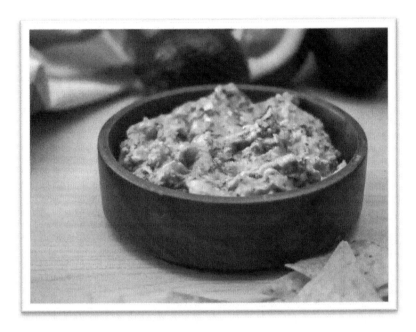

Preparation time: 10 minutes. **Total time:** 10 minutes.

Servings: 4

Ingredients:

- 2 medium ripe avocados, peeled, pitted, and chopped
- 1 small red onion, chopped
- 1 garlic clove, minced
- 1 Serrano pepper, seeded and chopped
- 1 tomato, seeded and chopped
- 2 tbsp fresh cilantro leaves, chopped
- 1 tbsp fresh lime juice
- Sea salt, to taste

How to Prepare:

1. In a large bowl, add avocado and mash it completely with a fork.
2. Add the remaining ingredients and gently stir to combine.
3. Serve immediately.

Nutritional Values: Calories 217; Total Fat 19.7 g; Saturated Fat 4.1 g; Cholesterol 0 mg; Sodium 67 mg; Total Carbs 11.3 g; Fiber 7.4 g; Sugar 1.7 g; Protein 2.3 g

Cauliflower Hummus

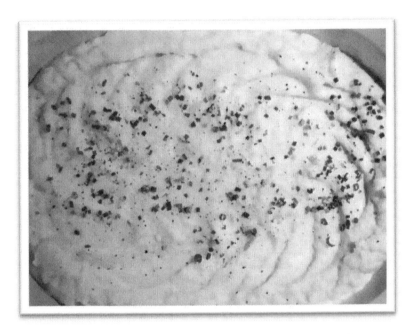

Preparation time: 15 minutes. **Cooking time:** 5 minutes. **Total time:** 20 minutes. **Servings:** 6

Ingredients:

- 1 medium head cauliflower, trimmed and chopped
- 2 garlic cloves, chopped
- 2 tbsp almond butter
- 2 tbsp olive oil
- Sea salt, to taste
- 2 tbsp fresh chives, minced
- Pinch of cayenne pepper

How to Prepare:

1. In a large pan of boiling water add the cauliflower and cook over medium heat for about 4-5 minutes.
2. Remove from the heat and drain the cauliflower well.
3. Set aside to cool it slightly.
4. In a food processor, add the cauliflower, garlic, almond butter, oil, and salt and pulse until smooth.
5. Transfer the hummus into a serving bowl.
6. Sprinkle with chives and cayenne pepper and serve immediately.

Nutritional Values: Calories 103; Total Fat 9.3 g; Saturated Fat 1.1 g; Cholesterol 0 mg; Sodium 63 mg; Total Carbs 4.5 g; Fiber 2 g; Sugar 1.6 g; Protein 2.5 g

Kale Chips

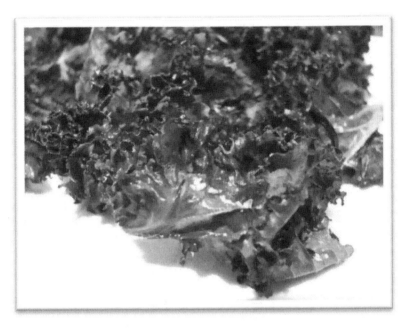

Preparation time: 10 minutes. **Cooking time:** 15 minutes. **Total time:** 25 minutes. **Servings:** 6

Ingredients:

- 1 lb fresh kale leaves, stemmed and torn
- ¼ tsp cayenne pepper
- Sea salt, to taste
- 1 tbsp olive oil

How to Prepare:

1. Preheat oven to 350 degrees F. Line a large baking sheet with parchment paper.
2. Arrange the kale pieces onto the prepared baking sheet in a single layer.
3. Sprinkle the kale with cayenne pepper and salt and drizzle with oil.
4. Bake for about 10-15 minutes.
5. Remove from the oven and let it cool before serving.

Nutritional Values: Calories 57; Total Fat 2.3 g; Saturated Fat 0.3 g; Cholesterol 0 mg; Sodium 72 mg; Total Carbs 8 g; Fiber 1.2 g; Sugar 0 g; Protein 2.3 g

Sweet Potato Fries

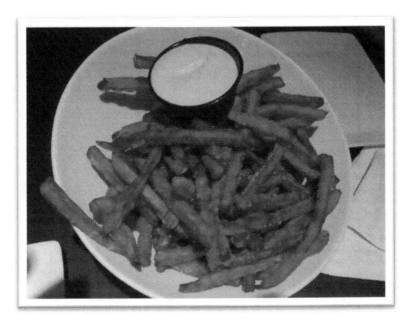

Preparation time: 10 minutes. **Cooking time:** 25 minutes. **Total time:** 35 minutes. **Servings:** 2

Ingredients:

- 1 large sweet potato, peeled and cut into wedges
- 1 tsp ground turmeric
- 1 tsp ground cinnamon
- Sea salt and freshly ground black pepper, to taste
- 2 tbsp extra-virgin olive oil

How to Prepare:

1. Preheat the oven to 425 degrees F. Line a baking sheet with a piece of foil.
2. In a large bowl, add all ingredients and toss to coat well.
3. Transfer the potatoes onto the prepared baking sheet and spread into an even layer.
4. Bake for about 25 minutes, flipping once after 15 minutes.
5. Remove from the oven and serve immediately.

Nutritional Values: Calories 199; Total Fat 14.3 g; Saturated Fat 2 g; Cholesterol 0 mg; Sodium 146 mg; Total Carbs 18.2 g; Fiber 3.5 g; Sugar 5.3 g; Protein 1.8 g

Seed Crackers

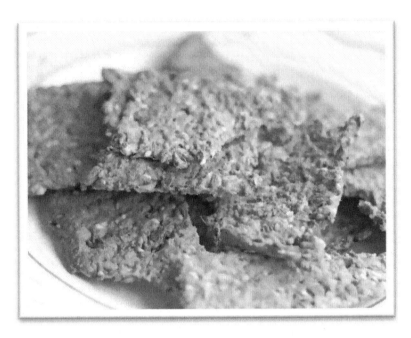

Preparation time: 15 minutes. **Cooking time:** 20 minutes. **Total time:** 35 minutes. **Servings:** 6

Ingredients:

- 3 tbsp water
- 1 tbsp chia seeds
- 3 tbsp sunflower seeds
- 1 tbsp quinoa flour
- 1 tsp ground turmeric
- Pinch of ground cinnamon
- Salt, to taste

How to Prepare:

1. Preheat the oven to 345 degrees F. Line a baking sheet with parchment paper.
2. In a bowl, add the water and chia seeds and soak them for about 15 minutes.
3. After 15 minutes, add the remaining ingredients and mix well.
4. Spread the mixture onto the prepared baking sheet.
5. With a pizza cutter, cut the formed mixture into desired shapes.
6. Bake for about 20 minutes.
7. Remove from the oven and place it onto a wire rack to cool completely before serving.

Nutritional Values: Calories 26; Total Fat 1.6 g; Saturated Fat 0.1 g; Cholesterol 0 mg; Sodium 28 mg; Total Carbs 2.5 g; Fiber 1.3 g; Sugar 0.1 g; Protein 1 g

Veggie Bites

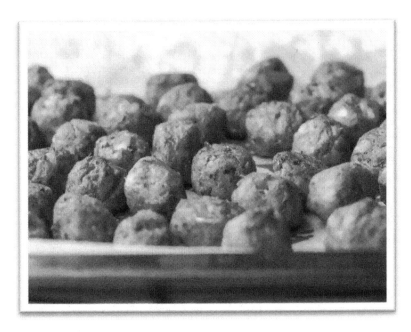

Preparation time: 20 minutes. **Cooking time:** 40 minutes. **Total time:** 1 hour. **Servings:** 6

Ingredients:

- 2 medium sweet potatoes, peeled and cubed into ½-inch chunks
- 2 tbsp coconut milk
- 1 cup fresh kale leaves, trimmed and chopped
- 1 medium shallot, chopped finely
- 1 tsp ground cumin
- ½ tsp granulated garlic
- ¼ tsp ground turmeric
- Sea salt and freshly ground black pepper, to taste
- Ground flax seeds, as needed

How to Prepare:

1. Preheat the oven to 400 degrees F. Line a baking sheet with parchment paper.
2. Arrange a steamer basket in a pot of water.
3. Place the sweet potatoes in the steamer basket and steam for about 10-15 minutes.
4. Place the sweet potatoes and coconut milk in a large bowl and mash them well with a potato masher.
5. Add the remaining ingredients except flax seeds and mix until well combined.
6. Make about 1½-2-inch balls from the mixture.
7. Arrange the balls onto the prepared baking sheet in a single layer and sprinkle with the flax seeds.
8. Bake for about 20-25 minutes.
9. Remove from the oven and serve warm.

Nutritional Values: Calories 135; Total Fat 4.3 g; Saturated Fat 1.5 g; Cholesterol 0 mg; Sodium 41 mg; Total Carbs 20.2 g; Fiber 5.3 g; Sugar 1.4 g; Protein 3.3 g

Roasted Pumpkin Seeds

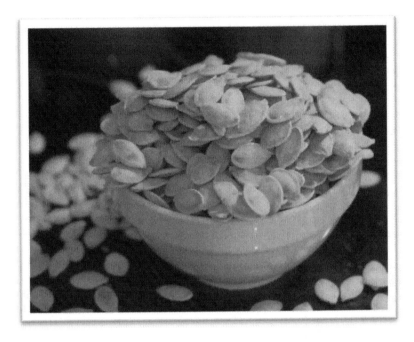

Preparation time: 10 minutes. **Cooking time:** 20 minutes. **Total time:** 30 minutes. **Servings:** 4

Ingredients:

- 1 cup pumpkin seeds, washed and dried
- 2 tsp garam masala
- 1/3 tsp red chili powder
- ¼ tsp ground turmeric
- Sea salt, to taste
- 3 tbsp coconut oil, meted
- ½ tbsp fresh lemon juice

How to Prepare:

1. Preheat the oven to 350 degrees F.
2. Add all ingredients except lemon juice to a bowl and toss to coat well.
3. Transfer the pumpkin seed mixture onto a baking sheet.
4. Roast for about 20 minutes, flipping occasionally.
5. Remove from oven and set aside to cool completely before serving.
6. Drizzle with the lemon juice and serve.

Nutritional Values: Calories 276; Total Fat 26.1 g; Saturated Fat 11.8 g; Cholesterol 0 mg; Sodium 69 mg; Total Carbs 6.4 g; Fiber 1.5 g; Sugar 0.4 g; Protein 8.6 g

10-Day Meal Plan:

Here is a 10-day meal plan made up completely of recipes found in this cookbook. Feel free to use it or create your own using it as a guideline.

Day 01

Breakfast: Quinoa Bread

Snack: Green Veggie smoothie

Lunch: Tomato and Greens Salad

Snack: Chocolate Milkshake

Dinner: Asparagus Risotto

Dessert: Baked Apples

Day 02

Breakfast: Tomato Omelet

Snack: Kale Smoothie

Lunch: Strawberry & Apple Salad

Snack: Strawberry Gazpacho

Dinner: Rice and Lentil Loaf

Dessert: Berries Granita

Day 03

Breakfast: Tofu and Mushroom Muffins

Snack: Grapes and Swiss Chard Smoothie

Lunch: Cauliflower Soup

Snack: Tomato Salsa

Dinner: Vegetarian Pie

Dessert: Pumpkin Ice Cream

Day 04

Breakfast: Blueberry Pancakes

Snack: Strawberry and Beet Smoothie

Lunch: Tomato Soup

Snack: Avocado Guacamole

Dinner: Green Beans Casserole

Dessert: Lemon Sorbet

Day 05

Breakfast: Bake Oatmeal

Snack: Peach Smoothie

Lunch: Garlicky Broccoli

Snack: Cauliflower Hummus

Dinner: Kidney Bean Curry

Dessert: Avocado Pudding

Day 06

Breakfast: Fruity Oatmeal

Snack: Papaya Smoothie

Lunch: Curried Okra

Snack: Kale Chips

Dinner: Black Bean Chili

Dessert: Chocolate Mousse

Day 07	Day 09
Breakfast: Spiced Quinoa Porridge	Breakfast: Chia Seed Pudding
Snack: Raspberry and Tofu Smoothie	Snack: Spiced Banana Smoothie
Lunch: Mushroom Curry	Lunch: Sautéed Mushrooms
Snack: Sweet Potato Fries	Snack: Veggie Bites
Dinner: Quinoa and Lentil Stew	Dinner: Lentil and Spinach Soup
Dessert: Blueberry Crumble	Dessert: Coconut Macaroons
Day 08	**Day 10**
Breakfast: Buckwheat Porridge	Breakfast: Nut and Seed Granola
Snack: Blueberry Smoothie	Snack: Oats and Orange Smoothie
Lunch: Glazed Brussels Sprouts	Lunch: Sweet and Sour Kale
Snack: Seed Crackers	Snack: Roasted Pumpkin Seeds
Dinner: Veggie Stew	Dinner: Vegetable Soup
Dessert: Apple Crisp	Dessert: Chickpea Fudge

Conclusion

With the information in this cookbook, it's hard to deny the importance of the Alkaline Diet. It can save you from the harms of acidic food and boost your metabolic activity by creating a suitable internal environment. The Alkaline Diet detoxifies your body decreasing your risk of life-threatening diseases.

The alkaline recipes here were created to give you innovative ideas for cooking healthy meals while maintaining proper pH levels. For more help following this diet, try the 10-day meal plan too.

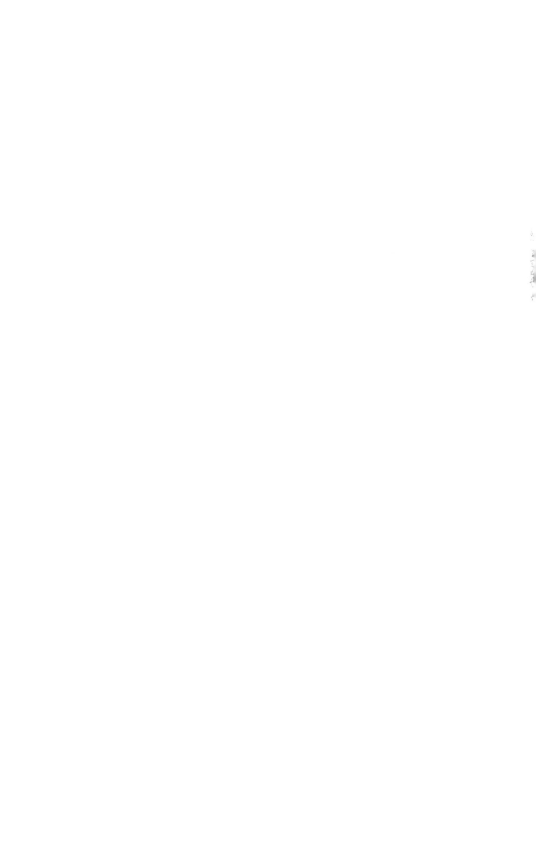

Made in the USA
Lexington, KY
21 September 2019